Additional praise for

Managing Anxiety in People with Autism

"I have had such great respect for Dr. Anne Chalfant for many years. She has a keen understanding of autism and has always offered tremendous insights in developing effective strategies to manage problematic behaviors and anxiety. This guide captures the wealth of her knowledge and experience for the benefit of us all. This is an essential resource for parents, caregivers, teachers, and professionals facing the challenges of autism."

—Sam Lo Ricco,
Founder and Chairman of Autism Behavaioral Intervention NSW,
and father to James, 10

"This is an accessible guide for how to understand and manage anxiety in autism spectrum disorders. It's written in a friendly, conversational tone and full of useful information."

—Lawrence Scahill, MSN, Ph.D.
Professor,Yale University School of Nursing and Child Study Center

"This book is a welcome addition to the bookshelves of many, many parents who have a child with an autism spectrum disorder. Parents will especially welcome the chapter on indirect treatments for use by parents, as well as the lucid descriptions of all treatment options available. The chapter on treating anxiety in parents and siblings of people with autism is also of great value. This is an easy-to-read book that is also scientific and precise, and the real-life examples from Anne Chalfant's caseload are interesting and hopeful.

With anxiety such a common feature amongst children and adults with ASD, it is marvelous to have a book which, for the first time, gives a comprehensive view of all the issues and all the treatments."

—Seana Smith, co-author, ***Australian Autism Handbook***,
mother of four children, eldest son has an ASD

Managing Anxiety in People with Autism

A TREATMENT GUIDE FOR PARENTS, TEACHERS, AND MENTAL HEALTH PROFESSIONALS

TOPICS IN AUTISM

Managing Anxiety in People with Autism

A TREATMENT GUIDE FOR PARENTS, TEACHERS, AND MENTAL HEALTH PROFESSIONALS

ANNE M. CHALFANT, PSY.D.

Sandra L. Harris, Ph.D., series editor

Woodbine House ◆ 2011

All rights reserved under International and Pan American Copyright Conventions. Published in the United States of America by Woodbine House, Inc., 6510 Bells Bell Rd., Bethesda, MD 20817. 800-843-7323. www.woodbinehouse.com

Publisher's note: The information contained in this book is not intended as a substitute for consultation with your child's healthcare providers. Although the authors, editor, and publisher made every attempt to ensure that the information in this book was up to date and accurate at the time of publication, recommended treatments and drug therapies may change as new medical or scientific information becomes available. Additionally, the authors, editor, and publisher are not responsible for errors or omissions or for consequences from application of this book. Any practice described in this book should be applied by the reader in close consultation with a qualified physician.

Library of Congress Cataloging-in-Publication Data

Chalfant, Anne M.
  Managing anxiety in people with autism : a treatment guide for parents, teachers, and mental health professionals / Anne M. Chalfant. -- 1st ed.
      p. ; cm. -- (Topics in autism)
  Includes bibliographical references and index.
  ISBN 978-1-60613-004-9
  1. Anxiety disorders--Treatment. 2. Autism in children--Treatment. 3. Family psychotherapy. I. Title. II. Series: Topics in autism.
  [DNLM: 1. Anxiety Disorders--therapy. 2. Child. 3. Adolescent. 4. Anxiety--therapy. 5. Autistic Disorder--complications. 6. Family--psychology. WM 172]
  RC531.C45 2011
  616.85'882--dc23
                                                                    2011015188

Manufactured in the United States of America

First Edition

10   9   8   7   6   5   4   3   2   1

In memory of my grandparents, Edith and John,
who taught me how to be "brave"
and in loving celebration of
my first born child, Frederick Anthony,
whose beautiful presence has helped put all my "worries"
into perspective and allowed me to focus on
what matters most, my family.

Table of Contents

PART III: DIRECT TREATMENTS FOR ANXIETY

Acknowledgements

Ironically, this book has been a source of "anxiety" at times. Trying to write a book, while managing other research and private practice commitments, has been a challenge. However, I have learned a great deal both professionally and personally in completing the book. The experience of writing the book was enhanced by the many people who contributed to the information and materials within it as well as those people who gave encouragement and support.

First, I would like to thank the families I work with who gave permission for me to include details from their cases in the examples throughout the book. These families are a source of inspiration in their courage and commitment toward assisting their sons or daughters with autism. Care has been taken to preserve confidentiality and privacy for all the families. In all instances, names and identifying information have been changed.

Second, I would like to thank my professional colleagues for their input. The team at Woodbine House has been insightful in their ideas and feedback regarding the book. I am also grateful to my colleagues, Professor Ron Rapee and Dr. Heidi Lyneham, at the Centre for Emotional Health, Macquarie University, Australia for their suggestions.

Third, my sincere thanks to my family for their enthusiasm and understanding throughout this journey. In particular, I want to thank my mother, Jeannette, and my husband, Justin, for their unconditional love and support.

Part I

What is Anxiety?

Introduction

The Purpose of This Book

Throughout my years of work and research, it has become more and more apparent to me that anxiety is one of the biggest challenges facing people with an autism spectrum disorder (ASD) and their families. In my practice as a child clinical psychologist, I have worked in a range of health settings, from large public hospitals to nonprofit organizations to private practice. Almost every family I see raises concerns about how to manage anxiety in their son or daughter. Similarly, almost every professional I work with asks about how to manage anxiety in his students or clients. Yet, despite the fact that anxiety difficulties seemingly go hand in hand with ASD, there is so little practical information available regarding how to manage it. I have written this book as a guide for parents and professionals to help fill the large gap.

The information in the book serves two purposes. Part I of the book provides a thorough explanation of what anxiety is, how it is experienced in people with an ASD, and why it seems to be so common. Parts II and III outline a range of practical strategies for parents and professionals to use to help manage and treat anxiety difficulties in their children, students, or clients with autism.

Anxiety in People with an ASD

Anyone who has ever experienced anxiety knows how crippling it can be. When anxiety is a problem, it can dominate the way you think; it can affect how you behave; it can change your appetite; it can disturb your sleep; it can lower your mood; and it can reduce your ability to carry out your daily tasks. For people with an ASD, life is already challenging enough without the added experience of anxiety to compound their difficulties.

Anxiety is considered an additional handicap for many people with an ASD. They can experience anxiety across all domains of their daily functioning including their school life, social life, and family life. Even the leading diagnostic manual that clinicians use, the *Diagnostic and Statistical Manual of Mental Disorders-Fourth Edition* (DSM-IV TR; American Psychiatric Association, 2000) highlights anxiety-like responses as a common "associated feature" of autism.

Why are people with an ASD so vulnerable to anxiety difficulties? First, we know that the core social difficulties in autism result in people with an ASD experiencing more social failures compared to other people their age, for example problems making friends or initiating play. As a result, they are much more likely to be anxious about their social abilities.

Second, we know that people with an ASD engage in "black-white," rigid, or rule-based thinking. This probably exacerbates any anxious beliefs they might hold. For example, if a child with an ASD once encountered an aggressive dog, then he might be much more likely than a typically developing child to believe that "*all* dogs are aggressive" and "*all* of my encounters with dogs will be with aggressive dogs." People with an ASD also have difficulties learning about categories and exceptions within categories. Therefore, the child in the example might be less able than a typically developing child to take on new information that represents an exception to his rule or belief. For example, he will be less likely to learn "some dogs are aggressive but most puppies are friendly."

Third, we know that people with an ASD have difficulty managing or regulating their emotions. Consequently, they are more prone to experiencing emotional extremes such as severe anxiety. People with an ASD seem to have difficulty identifying the early cues and triggers for their anxiety, and therefore controlling the rate of acceleration of their anxiety response. Consequently, in a feared situation, it is possible that someone with an ASD can experience a more accelerated anxiety response than another typically developing person.

Nowadays, when someone is diagnosed with an ASD, his family can access a range of intervention services to help target his difficulties with communication and social skills. For example, families are recommended interventions such as speech therapy, behavior therapy, early intervention play groups—the list is endless. However, I wonder how many times the issue of anxiety management is raised for parents at the point when their son or daughter is first diagnosed. I would hazard a guess that it is not raised frequently. Yet, while there is variation in the degree of communication and social skill difficulties for each person with an ASD, anxiety difficulties seem common to everyone with an ASD at some stage in their lives.

It is my strong opinion that we need to be more proactive in helping families and professionals better understand the role that anxiety plays in the lives of people with autism and in giving them skills to manage anxiety. To that end, even if your child has never shown signs of anxiety, there's no reason to wait until he might become highly anxious to implement the "indirect treatments" outlined in Part II of this book. The earlier you start to shift your parenting style to incorporate the techniques discussed in that section, the more resilient your child will be and the smaller the chance that your child will experience an anxiety disorder or problem. These days, intervention is all about addressing difficulties early rather than waiting until the problem is more obvious or impairing. The same applies to anxiety support. Parents who simply choose to incorporate some of the strategies described as a part of their parenting style, even if their child with an ASD has no worries or fears at all, will most likely find that they are helping to develop more resilience and self-confidence in their child.

How to Use This Book

This book contains descriptions and strategies that are designed to be both informative and practical. The first half of the book is dedicated to building your awareness of the anxiety difficulties of people with an ASD and their families. It aims to provide up-to-date information about anxiety, what it is, and how and why it occurs in people with an ASD. In Chapter 1, the main components of anxiety are outlined. The difference between helpful and unhelpful anxiety is explained along with how to recognize signs of unhelpful anxiety and the common types of anxiety disorders that people with an ASD experience. In Chapter 2, the reasons why people with an ASD are so vulnerable to developing anxiety difficulties are explored in detail. The variations in how anxiety presents in people with an ASD across different stages in their development are discussed in Chapter 3. Then, in Chapter 4, the impact of anxiety on the broader family of someone with an ASD is described. Ways that parents can inadvertently model anxious behavior for their son or daughter with an ASD are also discussed. By the time you finish reading the first half of the book, my hope is that you will have a good background understanding and awareness of the anxiety experiences of people with autism as well as the impact on families.

The second part of the book is dedicated to the treatment of anxiety difficulties. It contains strategies and tips for helping to manage anxiety in your son, daughter, student, or client. It also outlines formal treatment methods such as medication and cognitive behavior therapy (CBT). The strategies and treatments addressed are the latest, evidence-based approaches that have been shown through research to be effective in managing anxiety.

You will see that the second half of the book is further divided into two sections: one on indirect treatments and the other on direct treatments. "Indirect" treatments are the strategies that parents and professionals can use to adjust either their own behavior or the environment of someone with an ASD in order to reduce anxiety. They do not directly target anxious symptoms in the way that formal treatments such as medication or psychotherapy do. However, by changing behavior or the environment, these strategies will contribute to a reduction in anxiety for someone with an ASD. The strategies outlined for parents and professionals are similar in many ways. However, since home, school, and clinic environments are very different, it is important to look at each area separately. Consequently, separate chapters have been used to outline the strategies that might be helpful in reducing anxiety in each of these contexts. In Chapter 5, the book explores the strategies that parents can adopt to help reduce anxiety in their child and build his or her confidence. In Chapter 6, the focus is given to strategies that professionals such as teachers and healthcare professionals can implement to reduce anxiety in their students or clients with autism.

The "direct" treatments explored in the remainder of the book are formal intervention methods. They have been designed to target key anxiety symptoms such as the physical and mental symptoms associated with anxiety disorders. Direct treatments such as medication, psychoanalysis, and alternative medicine are reviewed in Chapter 7.

Cognitive behavior therapy (CBT) is reviewed in detail in Chapter 8 as are the other direct treatments available for anxiety difficulties. Finally, since the rate of anxiety difficulties is also higher in parents and siblings of people with an ASD than it is for families of typically developing people, Chapter 9 lists strategies for reducing anxiety in family members.

By the time you finish reading the second half of the book, my hope is that you will be able to select a wide range of strategies that you can apply to managing anxiety in your own son, daughter, student, or client with an ASD. There are some useful resources, books, and websites targeting anxiety management listed in the Appendices. These are provided in case you would like to follow up further with some of the key treatments and/or strategies referred to throughout this book.

Some Things to Keep in Mind as You Read This Book

Naturally, not all of the information or all of the strategies in this book apply to every single person with an ASD. Therefore, feel free to pick and choose from the book what is most relevant for your situation. Trial and error is often required when we try to treat a difficulty to make sure that the right approach is suitably matched to the problem.

You will notice as you progress through the book that a range of diagnostic labels are used including autism and ASD. In the book, these labels are not used to refer to different disorders. Rather, they are used interchangeably to refer to the same set of difficulties in social and communication skills, restricted interests, and repetitive behaviors. Therefore, the book applies to people with any ASD diagnosis including autism or autistic disorder, Asperger's disorder, atypical autism, and pervasive developmental disability not otherwise specified (PDD-NOS). Indeed, referring to these terms interchangeably seems even more appropriate now that we expect a new *Diagnostic and Statistical Manual of Mental Disorders* (DSM-V) to come out soon that puts forward new criteria where the one diagnostic label of autism spectrum disorder applies rather than a range of different diagnoses that represent different symptoms.

The information in this book is, of course, applicable to all children and adolescents with anxiety and an ASD, boys and girls alike.

To make the information more readable, I've alternated the use of gender by chapter.

For Further Assistance, Seek a Professional

Sometimes, people have severe and debilitating anxiety that requires more assistance than what can be provided from reading a book alone. In these cases I would recommend that you seek assistance from a trained mental health professional. There is a difference between reading information from a book and benefitting from the extra guidance of someone with formal training and qualifications in the area. To illustrate, although I read many books about pregnancy and how to prepare and make it through the birth of my first child, I still sought assistance from trained professionals including a mid-wife and obstetrician to ensure that I was correctly interpreting what I was reading. You will find that a trained mental health professional, such as a clinical psychologist or psychiatrist, will be well suited to assist you in using most of the strategies outlined in this book.

Will I See Progress and Will the Anxiety Go Away Totally?

You can certainly expect to have a better understanding of anxiety from reading this book. Consequently, if you increase your awareness of anxiety and how to recognize it, then you will be prepared to implement the strategies outlined in this book. You can also expect that the strategies listed in this book will be beneficial to most people with an ASD. However, you will need to adjust some strategies according to how significantly affected by autism the child is.

It is very important that you maintain realistic expectations regarding how quickly you might see a reduction in anxiety for your son, daughter, student, or client. Typically, progress occurs in a three steps forward, two steps back fashion rather than a ten steps forward and no steps back fashion. Sometimes you will adopt a strategy that makes life harder and feels like you are taking a backward step, before you see progress. It is important to persevere when you are working on managing anxiety. Usually, anxiety has been present for a long time and as the saying goes, "old habits die hard." There is no magic wand approach to treating anxiety difficulties in any individual. Like all good things that come to us, reduced anxiety is generally the product of hard work and effort over a long period of time.

Similarly, it is unrealistic and perhaps unhelpful to expect that all anxiety should go away totally. There is no one I know who does not experience some degree of anxiety in his life from time to time. Anxiety at a helpful level is a normal emotion that assists us in performing better and in achieving more. The aim of this book is to give you ways to manage and reduce unhelpful anxiety rather than eliminate all possible anxiety from life.

1 | **What is Anxiety?**

Justin and the Malouf Family

Justin was fifteen years old when he was referred to me by his school psychologist. At that time, both the school and Justin's parents were worried about his ability to make friends, his inconsistent academic performance, and his high level of anxiety in relation to both of these areas. They wanted to know whether or not there might be any underlying "problem" and, if so, how to help Justin. After reviewing the results of Justin's assessment, two main "problems," or diagnoses, seemed clear. First, Justin had autism. His early history, the school observations, and the formal diagnostic assessments that we conducted all seemed to indicate that he was someone with significant communication and social skill difficulties. He also had several unusual and intense interests compared with other boys his age. Second, Justin was experiencing Social Anxiety Disorder, otherwise known as Social Phobia. He presented with two fears particularly common to those with Social Phobia: fear that other people were evaluating him negatively and fear that he was always making a fool of or embarrassing himself whenever he interacted with others.

Even though Justin had autism and related social skill difficulties, there was no evidence to support his social fears of negative evaluation and embarrassment. He had not been teased or picked on by his peers. He had the potential to be an "A" student with a particular flair for English and he had not yet done anything at school to embarrass himself. Yet, despite the lack of evidence to support his fears, Justin seemed socially terrified. He avoided participating in class discussions even when he knew the answers (perhaps better than most of his peers) and he made regular visits to the school health room to avoid being with his peers during recess and lunch.

Of late, he had begun avoiding attending school altogether for fear that it might result in some kind of social disaster. Imagine the impact that Justin's behavior was having on his family life as he resisted attending school each day and became more and more aggressive in response to his parents' attempts to make him go.

When I met Justin he seemed shy and extremely nervous, rocking in his chair as we discussed his fears about school and his peers. Justin told me, "I keep thinking about what other people think of me." I will never forget some of his graphic descriptions regarding his feelings about socializing. He stated that he would rather "die from a lonely life than be humiliated." At another time he said that he would "rather be sliced up than have other people laugh" at him. He explained that his "brain goes blank" when he's with people his age and he ends up saying things that he believes are silly; e.g., "talking about a spleen and its properties and function in the body" when he draws a blank about what to say next in conversation. In summary, Justin had a range of social fears that were unfounded and over-exaggerated, however real they seemed for him.

Justin also described some physical changes he was experiencing whenever he was worried about school and socializing. He reported short-ness of breath, sweaty hands, racing heart, and nausea. Justin told me that whenever he noticed these physical changes he would start rocking and blinking quickly. He said that it was usually at this point when he would ask to leave the classroom and go the school's health room. If he was on the playground, he'd move away from the other children. Usually, he would end up in the school library. If there were too many people in the library then he'd call his mother and ask her to pick him up. When Justin came to see me, his mother was either taking him into school late or picking him up early from school several times each week. Mrs. Malouf's whole day seemed to revolve around waiting for "the call" to go and col-lect Justin from school.

Is Justin's Anxiety like that of Your Child, Student, or Client?

I could have substituted Justin's name with many other clients with an autism spectrum disorder (ASD) that I see for evaluation and treatment. We know that social anxiety is very common among young people with an ASD (e.g., Ghaziuddin 2002). The fear of negative evaluation, the physical symptoms, and the avoidance are all commonly reported to me by clients with an ASD.

Do you know someone with ASD like Justin? How many times have you heard of a child or adolescent with an ASD ending up in the school library at recess or lunch time because of social fears? Does your child tell you that she doesn't want to go to school because she doesn't know what to do and feels embarrassed or afraid? Does he ever say that he is too scared to speak to other students because he thinks they will laugh at him? Does your child avoid certain foods for fear of the taste or texture in her mouth? Does he place emphasis on completing his homework without any errors, doing it over and over again until it seems perfect? Does your son or daughter become anxious about sharing news, giving speeches in front of a class, or speaking at assemblies?

Does your student start to pace the room when something unexpected happens like starting the morning routine with math groups first when it normally starts with reading? Does your student ask repetitive questions to try to seek reassurance regarding *exactly* what will happen in math group, *exactly* how long it will take, *exactly* what materials she will need, and *exactly* how many questions she will be expected to answer?

Does your client insist on finishing his sessions early so as not to miss any of his Kung Fu class that follows because he's worried about missing out on an activity in the class and feeling confused? Consequently, does he regularly check his watch to ensure that the session is running on time and does he become increasingly agitated if it seems to be going even one minute longer than anticipated? Does your client have any phobias of situations like being at a noisy swimming pool because of fear of water or loud noises? Does your client have any animal phobias? If you answered "yes" to any of these questions, keep reading!

What Is Anxiety?

Typically, anxiety is defined as feelings of fear, apprehension, worry, or nervousness. People who have a "problem" with anxiety, otherwise referred to as an anxiety disorder, experience excessive levels of anxiety on such a frequent basis that it prevents them from carrying out their daily activities. In other words, these people are overwhelmed by their feelings of fear or worry.

Anxiety influences three key areas, 1) physiological (our body), 2) cognitive (our thoughts), and 3) behavior (our actions):

Physiological (Anxiety in Our Bodies)

We can experience a range of physical reactions in our bodies when we are anxious or stressed. These reactions occur because of a chain of events that happen automatically in our bodies when we face a situation that we perceive as threatening. The chain reaction is commonly known as the "fight or flight" response.

The Fight or Flight Response

The fight or flight response, also referred to as hyper-arousal or the "acute stress response," was first described by Walter Cannon in 1929. Cannon's (1929) theory states that animals (including people) react to threats with a general discharge of the sympathetic nervous system, which gets the animal ready to fight the threat or flee from it. How does this happen?

Without becoming overly technical, essentially, when a person is in a serene, unstimulated or calm state, the "firing" of neurons, or nerve cells, in the part of the brain that is involved with responses to stress and panic (called the "locus ceruleus") is minimal. However, when danger is perceived, there is increased "firing" of the neurons in the locus ceruleus making the person more alert and attentive to her environment. A more intense and prolonged firing of neurons in the locus ceruleus activates the sympathetic nervous system. The activation of the sympathetic nervous system is associated with specific physiological reactions in the system, through the release of the hormones adrenaline (epinephrine) and to a lesser extent noradrenaline. These hormones facilitate immediate physical reactions including:

- Racing heart
- Hyperventilation (see text box) and shortness of breath
- Turning pale or flush or alternating between both
- Digestion slowing down or stopping
- Constriction of blood vessels in many parts of the body
- Nausea
- Dilation of blood vessels for muscles
- Inhibition of a gland responsible for tear production and salivation, resulting in dry eyes and mouth

- Dilation of pupils
- Relaxation of the bladder, resulting in "accidents"
- Faster reflexes
- Shaking

So, when someone who is anxious faces a situation that she perceives as threatening, she experiences some of the reactions described above. Do you remember Justin's description of his experience of anxiety? He reported shortness of breath, sweaty palms, racing heart, and feeling nauseous. Justin was experiencing several physiological symptoms of anxiety.

What Is Hyperventilation?

Hyperventilation, or overbreathing, is the state of breathing faster and/or deeper than necessary. It brings about light-headedness and other undesirable symptoms often associated with panic attacks. Interestingly, the effects of hyperventilation are not related to lack of oxygen or air. Rather, by hyperventilating, we breathe out too much carbon dioxide, which reduces the carbon dioxide concentration in our blood to below its normal level. The reduction leads to constriction of the blood vessels that supply the brain and prevents the transport of certain electrolytes necessary for the function of the nervous system.

Cognitive (Anxious Thinking)

The idea that anxious people tend to think more catastrophically and negatively than non-anxious people has been long established (e.g., Beck, 1976). Anxious people have a thinking style wherein they tend to predict a negative or the worst possible outcome. Common examples of anxious or worried thinking include: "What if I make a mistake?", "I may make a fool of myself or do something embarrassing", "I'm not used to driving to the supermarket this way", "That dog could bite me!", "I have to get all of my spelling words right or else it won't be good enough", "The other kids at school might laugh at me."

People falsely believe that an object or situation causes us to feel worried or anxious. To illustrate, if someone sees a dog at the park that looks aggressive, she believes it is the sight of the dog alone that automatically leads to feelings of anxiety about the dog biting or attacking her. But this argument is flawed. Years of scientific research has taught us that it is not simply the sight of the feared object or situation that leads us to feel worried; rather, it is how we *interpret* the object or situation through our thinking or cognitions (e.g., Beck, Emery & Greenberg, 2005). That is, how we think about the feared object is what actually leads to anxious feelings, not the object itself. The two examples in Figure 1 help further illustrate this concept.

Fig. 1 | Thoughts Causing Anxiety

Example: A child gets up to deliver her news during "show and tell"
Thought: "What if someone laughs at me?"
Feeling: nervous or scared

Example: A child gets up to deliver her news during "show and tell"
Thought: "My news will be interesting."
Feeling: relaxed or confident

In the two examples in Figure 1 you can see that, in the same situation (a child preparing to deliver her news to the class), the child's feelings depend on how she thinks about or interprets that situation—not on the type of situation itself. It is the child's interpretation of the situation that causes her to feel anxious or confident. So, if we want to help that child feel better when getting up to give news to the class then we would not change the situation, that is, we would not stop her from presenting news to the class. Rather, we would try to change the child's thoughts or interpretation of that event.

Understanding that it is our thinking and not situations alone that affect our feelings allows us to see another means of preventing or managing anxiety. We do not need to reduce worry by avoiding a feared situation (e.g., talking in front of the class) or removing a feared object (e.g., dog). Rather, we need to change the way we interpret the situation in order to feel more confident towards it and "go for it!" It is the idea of changing negative or catastrophic thinking into more realistic or helpful thinking that underpins much of cognitive behavior therapy (CBT), which will be discussed at length in Chapter 8.

Go back to Justin's description of his thinking when anxious. He stated: "I keep thinking about what other people think of me," "I would rather die from a lonely life than be humiliated socially," and "I would rather be sliced up than have other people laugh at me." It was Justin's thoughts and catastrophic interpretations of his social experiences that were making him feel panicked and distressed, not the social experiences alone.

Behavior (Anxious Actions or Avoidance)

Anxious people tend to avoid the objects or situations they fear. Their avoidance serves to protect them from experiencing fear or anxiety. Moving away from the situation or object obviously makes them feel calmer and brings a sense of respite and relief. When anxious, we all avoid situations in many ways. Anxious people with autism are no different. Below are several examples of ways that people with autism might avoid a situation that provokes anxiety.

■ Refusing to start or to complete an activity in which they believe they might not succeed, for example class group work or a test. By avoiding the activity they ensure that they do not experience any possible distress or sense of failure.

■ Similarly, rushing through their work or tantruming during a challenging task in order to try to avoid working on the task.

■ Remaining in isolation on the playground rather than attempting to join a group of their school peers. By avoiding their peers they do not have to expose their social difficulties. That is, they do not have to try to read social cues, keep a social interaction going, initiate play; all skills that, by definition, are limited in children with an ASD.

■ Insisting that they get to school and any other appointments on time in order to avoid missing out on part of the activity or experience. In doing so, they avoid the possible sense of confusion. A client once told me that when he is late for his Kung Fu lesson he feels an acute sense of "confusion" and "frustration." Showing up late to a class made him feel that he would be "behind for the rest of the lesson." Therefore, he would avoid these feelings by insisting and even having a tantrum at home to ensure that his parents always took him to the lesson on time.

- Becoming physically or verbally aggressive (to themselves or to others) or running away in order to stop participating in a feared activity. One of my clients runs away from the classroom each time the workload becomes overwhelming and she feels that she might not be able to manage the task.

- Going to extreme measures to avoid any possible contact with an animal they fear. For example, a child I work with used to lock all the doors and windows in the house and then re-check the locks in order to ensure that the fruit bats in the trees outside did not fly into the house. (For those readers who don't live in Australia, fruit bats are very common here, but they are unlikely to ever fly into one's home!)

- Directing play with other children according to a pre-determined set of rules (often made up by the children with autism) in order to ensure that the interaction evolves according to their wishes. This prevents the game from changing form into something that the children with autism might be less familiar with or dislike and, therefore, less adept at playing.

- Sorting and repeatedly checking that their toys are all lined up in a particular order. Ritualized or compulsive behaviors such as checking and ordering are essentially a means for people with autism to avoid chaos or disorganization within their personal environments.

Avoidance can seem like a logical strategy for reducing anxiety. Indeed, many parents and professionals have suggested to me that avoidance is the best option for the anxious person with an ASD to quickly reduce her anxiety. Anxiety is an unpleasant feeling, and the desire to escape this feeling can be very appealing. For a personal example:

I feel anxious whenever I see a moth in my house →
I don't like feeling anxious → I avoid moths when I see them in my house →
I don't feel anxious anymore.

By avoiding moths, I teach myself that I am "safer" or I feel "better" away from moths. In turn, the next time I see a moth, I am more likely to avoid it than to face it because the last time I avoided it I felt better, quickly.

Some anxiety can be "normal" and even helpful (see section entitled "Helpful vs. Unhelpful Anxiety"); however, avoidance in people who are highly anxious is generally maladaptive. It has five main disadvantages:

1. Avoidance can erode confidence in the ability to face the feared or stressful object or situation.
2. Avoidance reinforces the idea that the feared object or situation is genuinely "bad" or "dangerous" and needs to be avoided, when it is usually quite safe or harmless.
3. Avoidance prevents us from having an opportunity to learn that a situation can be tolerated and might not cause anxiety.
4. Avoidance reduces confidence about facing other challenging situations, which in turn encourages further avoidance.
5. Avoidance that reduces confidence about our ability to handle challenges can ultimately reduce self-esteem and increase general feelings of insecurity.

Therefore, continued avoidance can reinforce and exacerbate existing fears as well as help create new fears. Consider the next example from a conversation I had with a client who is very fearful of dogs.

Child: *One day, I was in the front yard and I saw a big dog walking up the street. I think it was like a Great Dane; it looked like a small horse! It stopped outside our house when it saw me and barked really loudly. I saw its big teeth. It was so huge. I have never seen a dog that big. It was as big as me! I thought it was going to try to come into the yard and knock me over, bite me, or lick me. I've heard about that happening to other people. I freaked out, ran inside, and locked the door.*

Author: *How did you feel then?*

Child: *I felt better because I got away from the dog and it couldn't get me in the house.*

Author: *Did you ever see that dog again?*

Child: *Yes, I found out that it belongs to a family that lives a few blocks up the road. I saw it again a few weeks ago. Luckily it's so big that I could see it coming down the street from a fair distance so I managed to run into the house as soon as I saw it up the street, before it came too close.*

Author: *What about other dogs?*

Child: *I was at the park for a family picnic and some people came there to walk their dogs. I ran back to the car and sat in there until they left.*
Author: *Why? Was the dog from up the street there?*
Child: *No, but I'm not really used to dogs. It's possible that even small dogs could bark at me or run at me like the dog from up the road. I get really scared when I see most dogs now.*
Author: *What about dogs that are not real? What happens if you see a dog on TV?*
Child: *Well, there's this commercial on TV about breakfast cereal....*

What do you think happened next? Can you guess what the child said? Do you think she watches the advertisement? Or does she avoid it by changing the channel, turning off the television, or walking into another room?

In the example above, you can see how avoidance can make anxiety worse. The child shifts from avoiding one dog that barked to avoiding other dogs to avoiding images of other dogs (e.g., on television). Every time the child moves away from a dog, she is teaching herself that she is safer or feels better when she avoids dogs. The next time the child is near a dog, her anxiety automatically increases.

In this example, not only is the child's avoidance maintaining her anxiety about dogs, it is also increasing her anxiety about other situations where she might see a dog, real or in pictures. You can see how an unhelpful pattern of behavior starts to develop. This is the cycle of avoidance maintaining anxiety. If left untreated, the child's anxiety can lead to other types of possible avoidance, for example:

- avoiding the television in case she happens to see part of an advertisement about dogs;
- avoiding shopping centers where there might be pet shops;
- avoiding the outdoors in case she is in a location where people take dogs (e.g., parks, sports fields, her own street); and
- avoiding talking to people who have a dog in case the conversation turns to the topic of pets and then dogs.

As previously noted, one of the disadvantages of avoidance is that it prevents us from learning one very important possibility: that we might equally feel "safe" or feel "better" if we stay in the situation long enough to see that we can cope. In the example above, the child keeps running away each time she sees a dog. Her avoidance prevents her from learning that she might still be safe if she remains near dogs or watches the television advertisement.

Cognitive behavior therapy (CBT) (discussed in Chapter 8) deliberately targets avoidant behavior. From both research and the author's clinical experience, addressing avoidant behavior in people with an ASD can be the hardest but also one of the most effective areas of therapy for anxiety (Craske & Barlow, 1991). However, if we are going to help people overcome their fears about any object or situation, then we must allow them to learn the critical lesson that they can stay in the feared situation and cope.

Think back to Justin's description of his avoidant behavior when anxious. He stated:

- he avoided participating in class discussions;
- he made regular visits to the school health room to avoid being with his peers during recess and lunch;
- he had begun avoiding attending school each day, becoming aggressive in response to his parents attempts to make him go;
- if he was on the playground, he'd move away from peer groups, often retreating to the school library; and
- if there were too many people in the library, then he would call his mother and ask her to pick him up.

It was Justin's avoidance of school and social situations that made it harder and harder for him to cope at school because there were fewer and fewer opportunities for him to learn that he might be able to cope socially.

Helpful vs. Unhelpful Anxiety

Anxiety can be helpful as well as unhelpful. We have all experienced the sense of nervousness or worry before important occasions including a job interview, the first day at school, taking an exam, meeting someone new, giving a speech, competing in a sporting event, or awaiting important news from an anticipated phone call. We all need some anxiety to assist our performance in these situations. For example, when we prepare to take a test, we know that a certain level of anxiety and nervousness can enhance our performance. However, too much anxiety might cause us to panic and will affect our ability to effectively manage the task at hand.

How Can I Tell If My Child, Student, or Client Has Unhelpful Anxiety?

I would recommend using the following six key indicators or "red flags" to assist you in determining if your child or client is experiencing unhelpful anxiety and, therefore, if she is at risk of developing an anxiety problem or disorder.

1. *Frequency*: The anxiety is occurring regularly (i.e., on a daily basis or several times a day). For example, a child who is anxious every morning about arriving at school on time might be experiencing unhelpful anxiety.

2. *Type of object or situation causing anxiety*: The feared object or situation is one that might seem safe or harmless to most people. For example, it is reasonable and helpful to experience anxiety in response to the sound of someone trying to break into your home. However, it is less reasonable and unhelpful to experience high anxiety about the starting gun in a race at a school sporting event.

3. *Intensity of anxiety reaction*: When we experience an anxiety reaction that seems out of proportion to what the situation demands, we think of this as unhelpful. For example, distress like crying, screaming, tantrums, or aggression in response to a change in routine (e.g., a substitute teacher) would be considered intense and unhelpful anxiety.

4. *Degree of avoidance*: Going to extremes so as not to face the object or situation we fear is another indicator of unhelpful anxiety. For example, my client who would spend every lunch period in the school library so as to avoid the social experience of the playground was experiencing unhelpful anxiety.

5. *Can the anxiety be reasoned away?*: If it is difficult to try to talk someone out of feeling nervous or reason logically with someone when she feels worried, then her anxiety might be unhelpful. For example, when you cannot reason with a teenager by explaining to her that each time she gets in the elevator in her apartment building it is highly unlikely that it will malfunction and result in some kind of harm to her, then her anxiety might be problematic.

6. *Impact on daily living*: If the person or her family cannot carry out day-to-day activities because of the person's wor-

ries, then there is unhelpful anxiety. For example, when you can only drive your child to school using a certain route or she will throw a tantrum, then her anxiety is "unhelpful."

Helpful vs. Unhelpful Anxiety across Development

Table 1 depicts helpful and unhelpful anxiety at different stages in the life of a person with an ASD. Do any of the examples of unhelpful anxiety ring bells for you in relation to your own child, student, or client with an ASD?

Table 1	Examples of Helpful and Unhelpful Anxiety for Individuals with an ASD	
Stage in development	**Helpful anxiety**	**Unhelpful anxiety**
Infancy/early childhood	Occasional distress when a preferred toy or favorite unusual object is taken away.	Extreme attachment to a preferred toy/unusual object (e.g., sleeping with a favorite rock each night and carrying it around everywhere during the day). Tantrums and distress whenever the object is removed.
Childhood	Requesting to lead a social game to ensure that the rules are clear to other people playing.	Regular tantrums or hitting peers if they do not play according to the rules set by the child with an ASD.
Adolescence	Occasional worry about how to start a conversation with a peer group at high school.	Avoiding peers and retreating to the library or trying to leave school early each day.
Adulthood	Rushing so as not to be late for a meeting.	Repeatedly checking that all the clocks in the house are set to the right time so as not to be late.

In Table 1, you can see that the situations are similar but the reactions are different depending on whether the anxiety is helpful or unhelpful. It is the degree or intensity of the person's behavior, i.e., her level of distress or the extent of her avoidant behavior, that helps distinguish whether or not anxiety is affecting her daily life.

Types of Unhelpful Anxiety

As you might be aware, healthcare professionals, especially psychiatrists, pediatricians, and clinical psychologists, use the current diagnostic manual to determine what type of anxiety difficulty someone might have. Below are descriptions of some of the anxiety disorders that I see more often in people with an ASD.

Social Phobia/Social Anxiety Disorder: Fear of negative evaluation by other people. People with Social Phobia typically falsely believe that other people will laugh at them or think negatively towards them. Alternatively, they might erroneously believe that they are likely to embarrass themselves socially. Justin, in the case described at the start of this chapter, is an example of someone with Social Phobia.

Generalized Anxiety Disorder (GAD): Extensive worry regarding a range of issues including health, finances, family, future goals, current school or work, the state of world affairs, time, etc. People who seem to be constantly worrying about something are the kind of people that might fall into this category. Think of any children, students, or clients whom you know who worry excessively about their school work being on time, weather, crowds, current events in the world. It is likely that those people are experiencing GAD.

Specific Phobia/Simple Phobia: Fear of a particular object or situation and significant efforts to avoid contact with the object or situation. Some common examples of specific phobias I might observe in people with an ASD include fear of dogs, certain foods, colors, water, storms, and household objects that produce loud noises (e.g., vacuum cleaners or blenders).

Panic Attacks: A panic attack is not a "disorder" in itself; rather, it can be a feature of the physiological experience of any anxiety difficulty described herein. A panic attack is characterized by a sudden and rapid surge of intense fear or discomfort. The surge of fear involves at least four of the symptoms associated with hyperventilation described earlier in Chapter 1 (see text box) including:

- Palpitations, pounding heart, or accelerated heart rate
- Sweating
- Trembling or shaking
- Sensations of shortness of breath
- Nausea
- Feeling dizzy
- Chest pain or discomfort
- Chills or heat sensations
- Fear of losing control or "going crazy"

Obsessive Compulsive Disorder (OCD): Characterized by extremely intrusive thoughts (obsessions) that feel overwhelming for the person and cause intense anxiety. Usually, these thoughts are quite irrational and unrealistic. For example, one of my clients thought, "I could get sick and ultimately my family could become sick and die if any of the other students at my school touch me because they carry a virus." Given the intense anxiety triggered by obsessive thoughts, the person then feels compelled to engage in repetitive, ritualized behaviors (compulsions) in order to cancel out or neutralize the thought and, therefore, "prevent" (or avoid) the feared outcome. In the case of my client, she would avoid touching objects that were touched by the other students, remain in a special room in the school away from the students during recess and lunch, and refuse to bring school shoes into the house.

An Important Cautionary Note on OCD and ASD

In my opinion and based on my clinical experience, OCD is not as common in children with an ASD as is reported. That is, there seems to be a tendency to overdiagnose OCD in children with an ASD. Some professionals seem to believe that the third area associated with an ASD (i.e., the area of restricted interests and repetitive patterns of behavior) is characteristic of OCD and consequently they give both diagnoses. For example, children who engage in repetitive behaviors such as spinning wheels on toy cars, lining up trains, or sorting their toys over and over again into color groups might be diagnosed with both OCD and ASD because of their repetitive behavior. Similarly, children who have an ASD and impose rituals (e.g., insist that all the windows in the house must be closed to the same height) and become distressed when those rituals are not carried out are often given both an ASD and OCD diagnosis.

However, I believe that this kind of dual diagnosis might represent a misunderstanding of both the diagnostic process and the criteria. In other words, it is highly unlikely that many children who are given both diagnoses actually have OCD because their compulsive or repetitive behaviors are often not driven by anxiety. That is, it seems quite a leap in logic to assume that children with an ASD play repetitively because they are anxious. In the example of lining up or repetitively grouping toys, the children with an ASD lack imagination and creativity in their play. They tend to play with *parts* of objects rather than engage in more creative or pretend play with the *whole* object. They also have a strong ability to pay close attention to details (e.g., the wheels on a toy car) rather than focusing on the whole object (e.g., the whole car). Indeed, this tendency to focus in on details and object parts is a well documented characteristic of the thinking and learning style of children with an ASD (Happé & Frith, 2006). But these ASD characteristics do not necessarily occur because of anxiety. In my years of clinical experience, there seems to be little sense of the kind of "obsessions" that are required for a "true" OCD diagnosis in children with an ASD. Specifically, a child with an ASD might not necessarily want the windows of the house closed to the same height because of an intrusive thought that a parent will have a car accident if they are not. Rather, these behaviors seem based on a need for sameness and predictability in her environment rather than driven by some fear of pending danger or doom.

It is very important that we are clear about the differences between OCD and ASD, mostly because of the implications this has for treatment of children with an ASD. For example, if we are to overdiagnose OCD in children with an ASD, then we might also end up overprescribing certain types of psychotropic medication to help address problems that might not exist for these children. As we know, prescribing the wrong medication can be dangerous and, at times, life threatening.

Are There Other Aspects of ASD Symptoms Mistaken for Anxiety?

Stereotypical mannerisms and idiosyncratic movements (e.g., hand flapping, finger flicking, and other complex mannerisms) can be misdiagnosed as "tic disorders" exacerbated by stress and anxiety.

Anxiety can be a trigger for stereotyped mannerisms. However, for many people with autism, these stereotyped and repetitive behaviors relate more to sensory processing difficulties or to feelings of excitement and pleasure. Therefore, it is important to spend time determining whether or not a child's hand flapping is simply reflective of her having an ASD or whether it represents an entirely separate anxiety disorder that requires a separate type of treatment.

Current Statistics

Prevalence of Anxiety Disorders in People with an ASD

Prevalence rates of anxiety in children with an ASD offer some initial support to the argument that anxiety is a core difficulty of many children who have an ASD. Studies indicate that children and adolescents with an ASD experience a wide range of anxiety problems (Ghaziuddin, 2002; White et al., 2009). In fact, there is evidence that the rates of anxiety are up to four times higher in children with an ASD than they are in typically developing children. Most of the studies investigating the prevalence of anxiety in people with an ASD have suggested rates between 40 and 45 percent (Bellini, 2004; Simonoff et al., 2008; Sukhodolsky et al., 2008). However, several small studies have reported the prevalence of anxiety disorders in children with ASD to be as high as between 47 and 84.1 percent (Gillot, Furniss & Walter, 2001; Muris et al., 1998; Rumsey, Rapport & Sceery, 1985).

We know that anxiety occurs more frequently in children with high functioning autism than typically developing children. Now there is also evidence that anxiety difficulties occur more frequently in children with an ASD than they do in other groups of children with special needs. For example, it was found that children with an ASD present with higher rates of anxiety-related difficulties than children who have other neurologically-based impairments such as severe mental retardation and epilepsy (Steffenburg, Gillberg & Steffenburg, 1996). Children with an ASD have also been found to experience greater rates of anxiety difficulties than children who have a language disorder. When compared with children with expressive or receptive language disorders, children with ASD have been found to experience significantly more social worries, separation anxiety, and obsessive-compulsive symptoms (Gillot et al., 2001).

Table 2 gives some indication of the differing rates of anxiety in people with an ASD compared with the lifetime prevalence rates of anxiety for the general population as reported in the DSM-IV TR (American Psychiatric Association, 2000). From looking at Table 2 and from considering the scientific evidence we have from a range of prevalence studies to date, it seems logical to suggest that anxiety is a separate difficulty occurring over and above the symptoms of ASD. More importantly, on the basis of such high prevalence rates, it seems screamingly obvious that intervention programs that support the social and communication difficulties of people with an ASD also need to begin incorporating anxiety management strategies.

Table 2	Approximate Prevalence Rates of Anxiety Disorders for People With ASD and Without ASD		
Type of Anxiety Disorder		**ASD**	**Non-ASD**
Separation Anxiety Disorder		10%	5%
Generalized Anxiety Disorder		20%	5%
Social Anxiety Disorder/Social Phobia		40%	12%
Specific Phobia/Simple Phobia		30%	12%

Anxiety in Parents

Not surprisingly, parents of people with an ASD have also been found to have higher rates of diagnosable anxiety difficulties than other groups of parents. Studies comparing parents of typically developing children with parents of children with an ASD have demonstrated that the latter group tend to have fewer coping resources (Sivberg, 2002; Fombonne et al., 2001) and higher rates of anxiety and/or depression (up to 30 percent) (Fombonne et al., 2001; Piven et al., 1991; Wolf, Noh, Fisman & Speechly, 1989). More on this will be discussed in Chapter 4.

Gender Differences

Little is know about gender differences and anxiety disorders in people with autism. That is, we do not really know whether females with an ASD are more likely to have anxiety than males with an ASD. In the general population, we know that females are more likely to present with anxiety difficulties than males (McLean & Anderson, 2009). In part, this is because females are usually more likely to worry and ruminate ("chew cud") over their challenges (McLean & Anderson, 2009; Nolen-Hoeksema & Jackson, 2001), thus making them more vulnerable to negative interpretations of their experiences and to heightened anxiety. In my own practice I have observed relatively equal rates of anxiety difficulties in females and males with an ASD. Perhaps this is in part because although females might "worry" more, there are still more males than females that have an ASD and, therefore, there are more opportunities to view anxiety difficulties in them than might be observed in the general population.

Anxiety Assessment for Individuals with an ASD

Arranging an Assessment

Although a number of good assessment tools exist to help assess and diagnose ASDs, there are no specific standardized assessment tools designed solely for the purpose of assessing and diagnosing anxiety disorders within people who have an ASD. The best anxiety assessments that exist seem to be those used with typically developing individuals to determine the presence of an anxiety disorder. If your child, student, or client is to be assessed for anxiety difficulties, it is highly recommended that some of the following measures are used as a part of that process. Many of the assessments listed below are best administered by appropriately trained mental health professionals; e.g., clinical psychologists or psychiatrists. Generally, you might be best off finding a professional who specifically works with children with an ASD. However, most child clinical psychologists and child psychiatrists are well trained and experienced in assessing a wide range of children including those with an ASD. Clinical psychologists and psychiatrists typically belong to a professional organization. For example, in the US, most psychologists belong to the American Psychological Association (APA). Each organization has a website where parents can search for a psychologist with appropriate skills. For example, the "Find a Psychologist" link on the APA website allows parents to enter search criteria such as the specialist skills they are seeking (e.g., a professional who works with people with autism/PDD) and their local area in order to find the nearest and most appropriate professional.

Sometimes parents report to me that they feel a professional has not taken their concerns seriously enough by suggesting that the child's difficulties are "just the autism" and not specifically anxiety-related. The best way to try to prevent this situation is for parents to go to the appointment armed with detailed information about their child's anxiety, specifically referring to the three areas described above (physiological, cognitive/thoughts, and behavior/actions). The more detailed information that parents can provide about these areas and the level of intensity of their child's anxiety experience, the better able the professional is to understand the exact nature of the difficulty. If you see a professional who still does not take your concerns seriously after you provide them with this kind of detailed information, then consider getting a second opinion.

How can you tell if you have found a good clinician to conduct an assessment? In my opinion, a good clinician is someone who does the following:

- spends ample time with the parents, listening to their concerns;
- meets with the child or adolescent separately (depending on her age);
- observes the child in a clinical *and* natural setting if possible (e.g., meets with the child at the clinic as well as conducting a school visit to observe the child);
- speaks with other professionals working with the child (e.g., the child's school teachers); and
- uses some of the following measures as a part of the assessment process.

Structured Interviews

A structured interview is usually a consultation that occurs with the anxious person and her parents. During the interview, a list of standardized questions are asked to explore symptoms of anxiety. The interview helps determine whether or not the person's anxiety symptoms are consistent with the criteria for an anxiety disorder as outlined in the current edition of the *Diagnostic and Statistical Manual* of the American Psychiatric Association.

The Anxiety Disorders Interview Schedule for DMS-IV (ADIS) (Albano & Silverman, 1996) is one example of a structured interview schedule that is consistent with the DSM-IV criteria for diagnosis of anxiety disorders. Use of the schedule allows a trained mental health clinician to determine whether or not the person's anxiety-related difficulties might be severe enough to warrant a dual-diagnosis of an anxiety disorder and ASD. It can also help screen out other disorders.

Self-report Measures

Checklists and questionnaires can also be given to the anxious individual, her parents, and/or her teachers to complete. The measures provide insight regarding the specific symptoms that the person might have. They assess physiological and behavioral symptoms of anxiety as well as common worried thoughts that the person might be experiencing. The Revised Children's Manifest Anxiety Scale (RCMAS; Reynolds & Richmond, 1978), the Spence Children's Anxiety Scale (SCAS; Spence, 1998), and the Beck Anxiety Inventory (BAI; Beck, Epstein, Brown, & Steer, 1988) are all considered good self-report measures of anxiety. The RCMAS is designed for assessing anxiety in children, whereas the BAI is designed for assessing anxiety in older adolescents and adults.

Some measures include parent and teacher report forms to provide more information regarding their perceptions of anxiety and related emotional difficulties in the person as well as information regarding any challenging behavior that might be occurring. The SCAS provides a parent-report form to assess a parent's observations of anxiety in her son or daughter. The Strengths and Difficulties Questionnaire (SDQ; Goodman, 1997) and the Child Behavior Checklist (CBCL; Achenbach, 1991) provide both parent and teacher report forms for their perceptions of an individual's emotional difficulties. Finally, the Developmental Behaviour Checklist (DBC; Einfeld & Tonge, 1995) provides parent and teacher report forms that help to assess behavior and emotional problems in children, adolescents, and adults with developmental and intellectual disabilities.

Some of the measures noted above are accessed via publishers at a cost. However, some measures (e.g., SCAS, SDQ) are available for free online. (See Appendix A for a list of anxiety assessment resources and the websites where they are available.)

Cognitive Measures

For people with autism who are higher functioning (e.g., people with high functioning autism and Asperger's disorder), the use of self-report measures that look more closely at anxious cognitions might be particularly helpful in assessing anxiety difficulties. As explored earlier, anxious thinking perpetuates anxiety. Therefore, depending on the person's level of intellectual functioning, it might be important to determine what types of worries or anxious thoughts the person is experiencing. If we know the kind of anxious thoughts that a person has, then we are better able to tailor-make the treatment to target her specific worries or fears.

There are two good examples of self-report measures that target anxious thinking. The children's Negative Affect Self-Statement Questionnaire (NASSQ; Ronan, Kendall and Rowe, 1994) and the Children's Automatic Thoughts Scale (CATS; Schniering & Rapee, 2002) are both measures that look at anxious self-talk and negative self-statements. They cover cognitions regarding social threat (e.g., worries about other people laughing at you) and personal failure (e.g., feeling that you don't do things well enough). Both of these cognitions can be common within the anxiety experiences of people with high functioning autism or Asperger's disorder.

In Summary

- Anxiety generally presents with three components: physical, cognitive, and behavior.
- There is a difference between helpful and unhelpful anxiety.
- There are six key indicators that we can use to determine whether a person with an ASD is experiencing an anxiety disorder.
- There are alarmingly high rates of anxiety disorders in people with an ASD.
- Social Phobia/Social Anxiety Disorder, Specific Phobia/Simple Phobia, and Generalized Anxiety Disorder are common types of anxiety disorders experienced by people with an ASD.
- There is disturbingly little information about effective treatment of anxiety in people with ASD.

- We need to be careful that we do not overdiagnose anxiety disorders in individuals with an ASD.
- We also need to be careful that we do not misdiagnose characteristics of ASD as representing anxiety disorders.
- There are several good assessment tools that clinicians can use to conduct formal and thorough investigations regarding whether or not a person with autism has an anxiety disorder.

2 | Why is Anxiety a Common Problem for People with ASD?

Karl and the Potter Family

Mrs. Potter came to me with some concerns regarding her son, Karl, who has a diagnosis of atypical autism or pervasive developmental disability-not otherwise specified (PDD-NOS). Karl is ten years old and attends a local school where he is mainstreamed. His mother told me that this year Karl seemed to be spending much more time in the school library at recess and lunch time, away from his peers. Although the school reported to her that he seemed to be interacting with the other students in the library, for example playing chess or computer games, she expressed concern that he might be using the library as a means of avoiding social interaction on the playground. She further discussed that Karl had tried to make up health related excuses as to why he could not participate on the playground; e.g., that he was still recovering from a broken arm (that happened almost six months ago) or that he was feeling unwell and thought the library might be more relaxing in case it got too hot on the playground and he felt faint. He even complained about eye difficulties that might be exacerbated if he went outside in the sun. Naturally, Mrs. Potter had all of Karl's possible medical and physical ailments ruled out by their family doctor and some specialists before coming to speak with me.

Mrs. Potter indicated that Karl seemed to catastrophize how bad the social experience on the playground was. She reported that Karl would come home and tell her that his day was 10 percent positive and 90 percent negative because of spending time outside with his peers at recess or lunch. When she asked him why, he talked about a brief and *seemingly insignificant incident of another child throwing a ball in his direction and thinking that he was going to be hit by it and that the boy threw it at him on purpose.*

I also spoke with the special educator at Karl's school, who affirmed that Karl did seem to have a tendency to always see the worst in social situations even when they seemed harmless. She described one incident where Karl had misinterpreted and catastrophized someone's move in a chess game with him as a deliberate attempt to cheat in order to make Karl unhappy. In general, the rigidity in Karl's thinking and interpretations of social interaction was preventing him from engaging on the playground and feeling content at school.

Worries or "negative" thoughts are common in anxious children, whether or not they have an ASD. However, it is possible that children with an ASD are more predisposed to anxious thinking than other groups of children. Children with an ASD seem to have a natural thinking and learning style that is somewhat rigid or "black and white" (e.g., Rutter and Bailey, 1994). Interestingly, this is also the kind of thinking that we typically associate with a person who is anxious (e.g., Rapee & Heimberg, 1997).

How Does an Anxious Person Think?

Inflexible or "black and white" thinking has long been associated with the thinking styles of anxious individuals (e.g., Clark & Wells, 1995). It is argued that anxious people tend to process information in a restricted way. For example, researchers have shown that anxious children have a bias toward selectively attending to threat signals and, as a result, misinterpret ambiguous information as threatening because of a failure to consider the global context (Kendall, 1985).

Think of a flashlight. When you change the focus of the beam to hone in on an object, you can see a smaller area but you can see it in more detail. It is the same in the minds of anxious people. Typically developing anxious individuals tend to have a "narrow beam" that selectively illuminates what they feel anxious about in detail rather than also capturing information from the larger context that might reassure them that there is nothing to worry about. In other words, anxious people seem to have a bias for taking into account information that they consider threatening or fearful rather than taking other information into account as well (e.g., information about safety). For example, a typically developing child who fears getting injections, or shots, might have a bias toward thinking about all of the aspects of that situation that make him scared including the length of the needle, the possibility of pain during the injection, and the possibility of a foreign substance causing some harm in his blood stream. He is more likely to focus on this information alone rather than the fact that the needle is being delivered by an experienced nurse, that his parent is in the room with him for reassurance, that the shot won't last very long, and that it is highly unlikely that he will become sick from the injection. It is the child's tendency to over-focus on and over-interpret the "threatening" aspects of the situation that exacerbates his anxiety and doesn't allow him to consider the broader context.

Anxious adults also tend to engage in more black and white thinking styles. For example, if I am driving to a meeting and begin to worry about being late, I might limit my focus to the signals that highlight the threat of running late, for example checking my watch and the car clock, the people driving ahead of me who I believe aren't moving fast enough, and my over-interpretation that all of the traffic lights in the city are conspiring against me to turn red. I will probably not be thinking about the nonthreatening information such as how many times in the past I have driven the same route without running late, that the traffic is moving at a steady pace, that I am well prepared for the meeting, and that I can call ahead and let others know my status. Also, I might not remind myself that, if I am actually late, then the others whom I am meeting will more than likely understand as they know that traffic in the area is congested.

How Does a Person with Autism Think?

So, what is similar about the black and white thinking of anxious people and that of people with an ASD? Interestingly, like anxious people, individuals with autism have also been shown to have a "narrow beam" approach in terms of their thinking and learning styles. One prominent theory that helps explain this is the "weak central coherence" theory (Frith, 1989).

Central Coherence Theory

First proposed by Uta Frith (1989), central coherence theory refers to the idea that when we process information, we first explore the full or global context, and then we determine what out of that context is important to focus on in more detail. In other words, we use a wider beam on our "flashlights" to explore the bigger area, then we decide what information we want to adjust the beam over so as to explore more closely. Of course, these are decisions that are made in fragments of time. Thus we are unaware that we are going through that kind of thought process.

It is said that people with autism have "weak central coherence" (Happé & Frith, 2006; Frith, 1989). Specifically, people with an ASD have difficulty extracting meaning from a context due to a preference for processing local information first rather than global information (Happé, 1994; Happé & Frith, 2006). Instead of scanning the whole context in order to identify what is important to focus on, the person with an ASD is argued to be over-selective, focusing on small details and, therefore, less aware of other information in the environment (Happé & Frith, 2006; Frith, 1989). Going back to the analogy of the flashlight, people with an ASD seem to have a "narrow beam" focus on their flashlights, seeing less information but in greater detail. Therefore, some information remains out of sight since their flashlight beams are narrow and do not illuminate the bigger picture.

How often have you been speaking with a person with autism and heard him comment on a minute detail in a scene (real or in a picture) that you have missed completely and that does not seem particularly relevant to the overall image or point of discussion? For example, when I asked a client to discuss her day at school during our session she suddenly noticed and commented on the fact that she could see part of a cockroach's leg above the alarm system in the top left hand corner of the room. It took me some time to actually see what she was referring to and to realize that it was indeed the leg of a cockroach, which later crawled up the wall from under the alarm box.

Do People with Autism Have a Predisposition to Anxiety?

Do you notice similarities between the thinking styles of those people with anxiety and those with autism as outlined above? Both groups seem to take in information based on a "narrow beam" approach rather than processing information from the larger picture. On this basis, it seems quite reasonable to argue that people with autism might have an underlying predisposition to anxiety because they think in a similar way to people who are anxious. In other words, it could be argued that the weak central coherence of people with ASD might make them particularly vulnerable to anxiety because they might have a natural tendency to focus on threat cues rather than first processing the bigger picture, which would include non-threat cues.

Consider the example of a handwriting task. A person with an ASD who is anxious about handwriting might already have an underlying predisposition to focus firstly on the details of the task he considers threatening because of his narrow beam thinking style. Therefore, when a writing task is introduced in the classroom, he might automatically focus on where to write his name or on the pencil he is using rather than first taking in broader information such as what the writing task is about, how long the task will take to complete, and that he might have free time when the task is complete. Focusing on the aspects of the writing task that seem threatening could exacerbate that person's anxiety, making it harder for him to even start the task.

Similarly, in the case of Karl described at the beginning of this chapter, he seemed to have a bias toward focusing on certain details that he considered threatening and, therefore, to miss other important information in the "bigger picture." For example, he focused mostly on the ball coming toward him on the playground rather than trying to consider more global information such as the look on the face of the person throwing the ball, the game that person was engaged in, or the other people who were near the ball and might have knocked it accidentally in his direction.

Sensory Processing and Anxiety

Beyond their predisposition to black and white thinking, people with autism might also be predisposed to having more physiological symptoms of anxiety than other groups of people. All of us take in information and experience the world through our five senses, but for many people with autism, various sensations are felt more acutely within their nervous systems and can be a source of extreme physical discomfort. In fact, many people with autism experience fear and distress when processing sensory information. Indeed, for them, the mere thought of a pending sensation or sensory experience can result in extreme anticipatory anxiety (Ben-Sasson et al., 2008; Gal, Cermak & Ben-Sasson, 2007). Below are some quotes from parents of my clients or the clients themselves describing the intensity of their sensory sensitivities across the five senses.

Sensitivity to Sound: *"I don't like playing basketball in the gym. It is too noisy on the court. It hurts my ears. The echo when the ball is bounced makes me scared. So does the squeaky noise from everyone's shoes on the court. I can't concentrate on playing the game. All of the different sounds from the court become one big sound, like I'm standing in the middle of a thunder storm."*
—Mark, fifteen years of age with high functioning autism

Sensitivity to Taste: *"He won't eat any vegetables. We can't tell if it's the texture or the taste or both. We have cut them up into the tiniest of pieces and spoon fed him while he's watching television so that he is distracted when eating. But he'll dry retch, spit it out, or refuse to open his mouth."*
—John and Teresa, parents of James, five years of age with autism

Sensitivity to Touch: *"I can't wear certain socks or stockings. They make my legs throb. I also hate wearing my school jumper and some sweaters that must have a certain fiber in them, which makes me feel like a cat with all its hair standing up. I can't concentrate at all when I wear my school jumper. I just spend the day feeling itchy and aggravated because all I can feel is the way it rubs against my skin."*
—Stephanie, fifteen years of age with PDD-NOS

Sensitivity to Smell: *"He cannot tolerate the smell of meat. Obviously, I have tried cooking the meat in rich sauces like Bolognese with other strong smelling ingredients to disguise the smell but he complains that he can smell the meat and that it makes him feel nauseous. I have to make sure he is well away from the kitchen when I prepare anything that has meat in it. On the rare occasions when he eats meat, he has to hold his nose so that he doesn't become overwhelmed by the smell of it."*
—Tracey, mother of Zac, seven years of age with autism

Sensitivity to Sight: *"I avoid lights that are too bright. At home, I like to have all the lights in the house dimmed. When they are on full strength, it feels as though someone is flashing a light right into my eyes. It makes me squint and I get a headache. At school, I often get headaches. I always try to sit in the part of the classroom where there is less light."*
　　　　　　—Peter, ten years of age, with high functioning autism

In Chapter 1 we explored the physiological responses people have when they are anxious (e.g., rapid breathing, nausea, hyperventilation). These responses occur because of a chain reaction within the central nervous system. For people with autism, it seems that their central nervous system might be more frequently "stressed" because of their sensory processing difficulties. Consequently, they might experience the physiological symptoms of anxiety more frequently than other people.

In Summary

- Anxious individuals seem to have a tendency to focus first on threatening information rather than the broader context including nonthreatening information.
- People with autism seem to have an underlying tendency to focus on specific details rather than the broader context. We refer to this as "weak central coherence" or a "narrow beam" thinking style.
- There is a striking similarity between the "narrow beam" thinking style of people with an ASD and the tendency of people with anxiety difficulties to focus selectively on threat-based information.
- The resemblance in the thinking styles of these two groups of people suggests that individuals with autism are likely to be more susceptible to anxiety because they more naturally think like anxious people.
- People with autism tend to experience sensory processing difficulties that can lead to anxiety in anticipation of a sensory experience.
- Since sensory processing difficulties are more common in people with autism, then people with an ASD are

more likely to be vulnerable to higher anxiety than other groups of people.

3 | Anxiety across the Stages of Development

Mitchell, aged six

Mitchell's mother reported that Mitchell had "another meltdown" at school this week over the class toy. It was a plush toy version of the school mascot and it was being used as a part of a classroom reward system. Essentially, the student who earned the most points would be able to take the toy mascot home over the weekend as a special treat. The reward system had been implemented approximately three weeks ago and Mitchell had not yet earned enough points to be the chosen child. When Mitchell's mother mentioned this to our staff, both she and our team agreed that it was yet another example of Mitchell's challenge with coping when he is not the "winner," not the person coming first, nor the one considered the best student. Mitchell would run out of the classroom every week after the mascot winner was announced. Moreover, when picked up from school he would cry and tantrum for up to thirty minutes. Mitchell's mother also reported that from the start of each school week Mitchell was spending much of his time worrying about earning mascot points, tracking the mascot points earned by each class member, and becoming anxious if he determined that he was lagging behind in the points being earned.

Robin, aged thirteen

Robin worried about socializing with people her age. She spent most lunch times in the school library or wandering alone on the playground. Despite evidence that her peers actually liked her and would try to include her in their play or activities she seemed to avoid social contact with them beyond the classroom. Robin said that much of the time she worried that her peers thought she was "weird." As a result of this she also thought that *if she tried to socialize with them, then they would most likely laugh at her or tease her. She seemed constantly worried about making a fool of herself in front of them, despite their seeming genuinely interested in her.*

Robin's mother had noticed that her worries about socializing at school were starting to affect her responses to other people when they made social overtures toward her. For example, she described an incident of a child approaching Robin one lunch time to speak with her about a computer game they were both interested in. However, because of her anxiety, Robin reportedly thought that the boy must have been trying to use the game as a way of teasing her about her strong preference for computer games over other activities. Consequently, Robin had become defensive and dismissive of the boy, giving one word answers rather than keeping the conversation going.

Geoff, aged fifty-three

Geoff accompanied his twenty-one-year-old son to see me regarding getting support for his son with social skills. However, as their initial consultation progressed and I took some information from both gentlemen about their family history and background, Geoff began to cry. He stated that he believed he had high functioning autism, that he was highly anxious and not coping. He described many worries regarding whether or not he had provided enough as a father for his children and whether or not he was a good husband. Also, he worried that he was underachieving in his life and that his family resented him. Often, he felt inadequate, as though everything was "hopeless." Geoff described worrying about these issues constantly. It seemed clear that his self-esteem and mood were particularly low. He also discussed that he was not eating well, was not sleeping well, and could not concentrate at work. Geoff described that he felt constantly anxious at work. When trying to fall asleep each night, he would spend time worrying about how to "do better" in his work and within the family. It seemed that Geoff's anxiety was so impairing that he was also suffering with clinical depression. Indeed, Geoff indicated that he had contemplated suicide on several occasions.

Autism and the Stages of Development

Our development is characterized by a range of cognitive, social, and emotional markers, or steps. Over the years many developmental psychologists have demonstrated that these markers might be thought of as set "stages in development." For example, the famous philosopher and developmental psychologist Jean Piaget suggested four stages of cognitive development in children (e.g., Piaget & Inhelder, 1973) while equally renowned developmental psychologist and psychoanalyst Erik Erikson proposed a theory of eight stages of social development across the life span (e.g., Erikson, 1950). Nowadays, if you walk into a bookstore and pick up any parenting book or book on childhood, you will find almost all of them outline stages regarding what to expect of children at various ages in terms of their behavior, their social skills, and their emotional development.

However, as we know, autism is a *developmental* disorder. This means that autism can impact on the normal development of a person's cognitive skills, communication skills, social skills, emotional awareness, and resilience. But interestingly, the reverse also applies: autism is affected by the developmental stages each person goes through. That is, the presentation of autism in a person seems to change as the person matures and develops. For example, the unusual preoccupations with sticks that we might have observed in a preschooler with autism might be replaced by an intense or obsessive interest in dinosaurs as the child gets older, which might be later substituted with a preoccupation with public transportation when the child reaches adolescence.

Therefore, anxiety in people with autism also changes as the person moves from one stage of her development to another. For example, young children with autism are more likely to experience anxiety about boundaries, limits to their behavior, and changes in routine, whereas adolescents with autism are more likely to experience anxiety about social difficulties and fitting in with their peer group. From the previous examples of Mitchell, Robin, and Geoff, you can see that each one is experiencing high anxiety. However, they are experiencing their anxiety in different ways and in relation to different content because Mitchell, Robin, and Geoff are all at different stages in their development. That is, the source or content of someone's anxiety difficulties is likely to change as they grow and mature.

It is helpful to try to understand how and why anxiety presents differently across the developmental stages of someone with an ASD. Knowing what key signs to watch out for might be beneficial for parents, teachers, and professionals working with people with autism. If we can better recognize possible signs of anxiety at each stage of an individual's development, then we can act sooner and more effectively in assisting the anxious person with autism. The longer anxiety difficulties are left without intervention, the harder they are to treat and the greater the risk of other difficulties arising such as depression. Consequently, the next section of this chapter takes a much closer look at each stage of development and how autism affects it. The chapter then explores how the anxiety difficulties of someone with an ASD might change across the age ranges. A good summary of this information is also provided for your reference in Table 3.

Anxiety in Children with Autism

What Are Some of the Key Characteristics of "Normal" Child Development?

Developing a Secure Attachment to the Parent

Through shared experiences, affection, and nurturing, the parent-child bond is strengthened. Children learn that they can trust their parents. They develop a sense of pleasure from showing preferred toys to parents, pointing items out to parents, and sharing a play experience with their parents. They also spend time watching their parents and imitating them. Parents usually see themselves in their children's behavior, for example when children copy the way parents talk on the phone.

Understanding Boundaries to Behavior

By testing limits, children are able to learn what boundaries will be placed on their behavior by their parents. We see this demonstrated during the period often referred to as the "terrible twos," when typical development is often characterized by tantrums and challenging behavior. Only last night while having dinner with my two-year-old cousin and our family did I see an example of such challenging behavior. My little cousin removed herself from the dinner table, walked to the couch, and asserted to the group of adults with a smile, "I am on the naughty chair because I'm not eating my dinner." She seemed to be waiting for attention and a limit to be asserted by an adult in the group. It is by engaging in this kind of challenging and attention-seeking behavior that children come to understand what parents deem acceptable or unacceptable and, therefore, how to adjust their own behavior accordingly.

Imaginative Play and Play with Other Children

In childhood, we see the development of creativity in play. Children develop skills to use objects to represent other objects (e.g., to pretend that a block is a train). They also develop the ability to vary their play creatively, for example taking a doll to the park one day, then having a tea party with the doll the next day. In the preschool years, children begin to develop skills in social play. They begin to learn about initiating social interaction with other children by approaching them and initiating play with them, by showing another child a toy, or by sharing a toy via turn taking.

Learning More Formal Rules and Academic Skills

Later in childhood, particularly during the elementary school years, children develop an understanding of societal rules (e.g., to wait your turn when someone else is speaking, to listen to and generally comply when an adult gives you an instruction). They also develop foundation academic skills in literacy and numeracy, which form the basis for their learning and abstract reasoning for the rest of their lives.

How Does Autism Affect These Stages of Child Development?

Challenge to Developing a Secure Attachment

Autism challenges children's ability to develop a secure attachment to their parents. We know that in autism, children tend to have difficulty initiating joint attention with their parents. That is, they struggle to share an experience with their parents. For example, many children with autism do not point out preferred objects to their parents or bring their parents a favorite toy to show them what happens when it's played with. We also know that children with autism seem to watch and imitate their parents' behavior much less than typically developing children. In addition, they have difficulty responding to their parents when their names are called. These challenges of poor joint attention, limited pointing, limited showing, reduced imitation, and limited response to name are often referred to as the "red flags" of autism. They are considered the early warning signs that something might not be quite right with a child's development because the child is not developing the characteristics we would expect to see in her early childhood.

Challenge to Understanding Boundaries

Autism challenges children's ability to understand boundaries for their behavior. It is often said that children with autism seem to be "in their own world." They are noted to have difficulty taking on other people's perspectives and, therefore, accepting boundaries and limits that might be placed on them by other people, especially their parents. Indeed, parents might typically find that it is not enough to say "no" or "stop" to a child with autism. Rather, they might have to use extra aids such as visual supports and social stories to help their child understand what is and is not acceptable behavior.

Challenge to Imaginative Play and Social Play

Autism challenges creative play in childhood. Children with autism tend to engage in repetitive use of toys and objects and to explore them by their properties. For example, they might repetitively watch how a toy car door opens and shuts rather than drive it to an invented location (e.g., driving the car to the pretend gas station and pretending to put gas into the toy car). The tendency of children with autism to have restricted play interests and repetitive ways of interacting with objects seems to stifle the development of imaginative play.

Moreover, autism challenges social play. Indeed, we consider limited social skills to be among the core deficits of children with autism. Their tendency to be rigid in their thinking and to have a narrow range of interests affects their ability to follow or share in the interests of other children their age. Consequently, they might not approach other children their age to engage in shared play. Moreover, they might have significant difficulties taking turns and sharing objects with other children unless those children are prepared to play according to the rules set down by the children with an ASD.

Challenge to Learning Formal Social and Academic Skills

Autism challenges children's ability to understand and accept some societal rules often first taught and experienced in the elementary school years. Basic classroom social skills such as waiting for your turn, keeping your hands to yourself (even when frustrated), participating in group activities, and respecting and following adult instruction can be challenging for children with autism. They might insist on sameness in their routines, including always being first in a line or always being able to win a class game or activity. They might prefer not to participate in group activities because of their limited social skills. They might have difficulty complying with adult instruction, preferring to follow their own choices or ideas.

Elementary or grade school is usually a time to learn about teams and develop skills to participate on teams. For example, there is typically a heavy focus on participation in team sports. However, for children with autism, their limited social and, at times, weaker motor coordination might challenge how well they can participate in any team, especially team sports.

Autism also affects children's ability to follow academic tasks and develop key academic skills in literacy and numeracy. For example, the language and communication impairments associated with autism can make it difficult for children to process large amounts of auditory information and complete tasks that tap into their weaker developed language and communication skills including reading, spelling, and written expression. Consequently, some of these foundation learning skills can be delayed or impaired.

What Are the Common Signs of Anxiety in Children with Autism?

Signs of Anxiety in Early Relationship Development

Given the difficulties with joint attention of young children with autism, we might assume that, in general, they would feel more comfortable "in their own world." They might be happier left to their own devices rather than interacting with a parent. It follows then that when adults make attempts to engage the child by repeatedly calling her name, shifting the child's face to capture eye contact, or bringing toys to the young child to try to engage her in shared play, it might lead to stress and anxiety for the child. Of course, no parent tries to make their child feel anxious. Moreover, for parents, the lack of response from their own child towards them must be heart-breaking. However, think of the anxiety for a young child who does not have the skills to respond to her name, or share in play with the parent when the parent repeatedly prompts or even physically tries to force the child into interaction. Acts such as taking a preferred toy away until the child looks at the parent, interrupting the child's play, or picking up her preferred toy or object and playing with it to see if the child will respond can exacerbate the child's anxiety.

So many parents I work with report intense emotional responses from their child when they interrupt their child's individual play to redirect her away from a solitary activity to one that includes the parent, for example re-directing the child away from lining up trains to setting up a pretend tea party. Commonly reported indicators of anxiety in early relationship development might include:

- crying,
- screaming,
- dropping to the floor,
- tantrums,
- throwing objects,
- hitting the parent, or
- self-harming (e.g., biting, head banging, pulling her own hair or eyelashes).

If a child with autism becomes anxious about interaction outside of her own interests, then it is possible that this anxiety will affect the strength of the relationship that develops between her and her parents. To address this problematic possibility, many recently devel-

What is Child-Directed Play?

Child-directed play is essentially following your child's lead during play rather than trying to direct her. During child-directed play, the parent gives undivided attention to the child by closely observing and commenting on what the child is doing, for example, "Oh wow, I see you've used the blocks to build a tower..." rather than making suggestions for the child to follow or incorporate into her play. The quality of attention that the child receives from her parent during child-directed play is very rich because the parent follows the child's agenda and uses the time to observe the child on the child's terms. Consequently, regular child-directed play is argued to help foster more a positive relationship between the parent and child and to have indirect benefits for the child's self-confidence and self-esteem.

oped methods of early intervention have shifted focus. They now aim to encourage parents to spend more time following their child's lead and entering the "child's world" during play rather than encouraging the child with autism to "enter the parents' world." In psychology, this is referred to as child-directed play.

Signs of Anxiety in Early Play

It has been argued that children with an ASD have a tendency to engage in repetitive or nonfunctional behavior because it helps to provide a sense of self-soothing, order, or predictability in contrast to the chaos and unpredictability they might feel during social interaction. That is, repetitive behavior might have a stress-reducing function (e.g., Lewis & Bodfish, 1998). For example, a parent reported to me that she can tell when her son is anxious about entering a social situation because he begins to pace back and forth and "mouth" his shirt. Perhaps not surprisingly then, other signs of anxiety in early development can include an increase in stereotyped behavior and repetitive language. Common behaviors that indicate anxiety in early play might include:

- lining up toys or objects (e.g., lining up dolls);
- repetitively stacking and knocking over objects (e.g., blocks);
- collecting objects or parts of objects (e.g., bottle tops);
- sorting toys or objects into groups by color, shape, or size;
- echolalia or repeating phrases out loud (e.g., quoting the same phrase from a movie repetitively);
- repetitively moving objects or object parts in the same way (e.g., pushing a button on a toy over and over to hear it make the same sound);
- repetitive movements (e.g., tic-like movements such as facial grimacing); or
- repetitive hand and arm movements (e.g., hand-flapping).

Signs of Anxiety in Social Interactions with Other Children

Children with an ASD might become anxious when play does not unfold as they want or expect it to. Typically, they seem to fear another child joining their game and making new suggestions, which might change the rules. Even worse might be the common occurrence of other children choosing to play a completely different game altogether. The best way for a child with an ASD to stop this from occurring is either to play alone or to try to control or "police" the other children with whom they chose to play. Therefore, common signs of anxiety in play with other children might include:

- earnestly allocating herself as "the boss" of the game (e.g., "I'm the leader and you have to do what I say.");
- scripting play for other children (e.g., "You say/do...then I'll say/do...") if playing creatively to ensure that there is no deviance from the "script";
- showing frustration when the play shifts from the original "plan" by having a tantrum, yelling, hitting, or throwing an object;
- avoiding social play altogether (e.g., wandering alone on the playground); or
- interrupting other children's play and removing the object they are playing with (e.g., running into a soccer game and taking the ball away).

Signs of Anxiety in Formal Schooling Years

Children with autism seem to rely heavily on sameness in their routines especially in their elementary school years. They are usually the ones most familiar with the order of activities during the day, the classroom rules, the teacher's common expressions, and the procedures associated with group activities. For children with autism, it is important that there is little variation in their daily school experience, unlike other children for whom change helps create diversity and stimulates interest in learning. When change occurs, children with autism might become challenging to teach. Unfortunately, sometimes teachers find the challenging behavior of children with autism an indication of an oppositional or defiant personality, precociousness, rudeness, or lack of respect. However, more than likely, challenging behavior can be a sign of the extent of the children's anxiety or worry. Common signs of anxious behavior during the elementary school years might include:

- correcting the classroom teacher,
- refusing to participate in a "new" task,
- running away,
- having a tantrum in the classroom,
- trying to take over and rearrange the schedule back to the way the child prefers it, or
- bargaining, negotiating, or even arguing with the teacher.

It is important to bear in mind that these signs of anxious behavior can also be seen in typically developing kids or be signs of other difficulties, e.g., learning difficulties. Therefore, a closer look at the purpose of the behavior (i.e., using a functional behavior analysis, or FBA) might be useful. Many helpful books exist on this subject, including *Functional Behavior Assessment for People with Autism* by Beth A. Glasberg (Woodbine House, 2006).

Anxiety in Adolescents with Autism

What Are Some of the Key Characteristics of "Normal" Adolescent Development?

Developing a Sense of Independent Identity and Autonomy

By the time a child reaches adolescence, she has begun to see herself as a "young adult." She sees herself less as a "minor" member of the family, who must simply accept and follow parental suggestions and choices including rules, and more of an equal to her parents in terms of the family hierarchy. It follows that she often believes she is as able as her parents to start making her own choices and decisions on issues that her parents may once have had final say over. I am sure we have all encountered that phase in development when suddenly the teenager begins to have more say in relation to what she will/won't eat, what she will/won't wear, when she will/won't come home from a social event, which friends she will/won't associate with, or when she will/won't study or complete homework. Most parents find the period of adolescence extremely difficult to navigate. They struggle to work out the right balance between when to become more flexible to allow their teenager to develop her own sense of identity and when to continue to set limits and boundaries for their teenager's protection and longer term happiness.

It is also at this stage that adolescents start to become more autonomous or self-sufficient. For example, many decide to take on casual weekend jobs for extra spending money. Others start to make decisions about their longer term careers, for example teenagers who leave school early to take on apprenticeships and trades. They also start to become more self-sufficient in directing their own learning, including planning and organizing their own homework, assignment completion, exam preparation, and study.

Risk Taking and Rebellion

Unfortunately for parents, the adolescent years are full of periods of limit testing and risk taking. At times, adolescents develop a sense of infallibility because they are at a developmental stage where they feel old enough to engage in adult activities, e.g., driving, drinking alcohol, engaging in sexual behavior, and even experimenting with drugs. However, developmentally, they are not yet mature enough to plan ahead for the possible longer term consequences of such risk taking behavior. In going against the norms and rules, adolescents are trying to assert their independence and experiment with various social rules in order to best determine which ones fit them.

Associating More with Peer Groups and Less with the Family Unit

I'm sure you have heard many a parent say, "She hardly talks to me now. I get one word answers or grunts. She talks more to her friends than she does to me." Parents who have reported this to me are highlighting the typical transition of an adolescent away from the family unit and toward her peers. We have all experienced times when adolescents seem like they would like to spend more time with their friends than at home with the family. They might ask to stay home when family outings or vacations are planned. Perhaps they hardly talk about their day at school but then spend hours on the phone with a classmate. In general, the typical adolescent years are full of socializing more with other people the same age and less within the family.

How Does Autism Affect these Stages of Adolescent Development?

Challenge to Developing Independence and Autonomy

Teenagers with an ASD are likely to become more dependent on their parents as the social and learning demands associated with adolescence increase. They seem to make the opposite transition than their typically developing peers. While typically developing teenagers start to develop their own self-sufficiency, the limited social insight, poor planning, and organization difficulties associated with autism make it hard for these individuals to understand that they must take a more active role in looking after themselves (McGovern & Sigman, 2005). They struggle to think about or understand concepts such as seeking casual work to earn their own money, developing and following their own study schedules, and taking care of their own personal hygiene and physical appearance.

I recall two concerned parents who came to see me about this very problem for their sixteen-year-old son with autism. They were trying to teach him to become more self-sufficient by helping him seek casual work in either the local library or a video shop (both of these choices related to his interest and knowledge areas in nonfiction reading and movies). However, it was clear to me when I met with their son, Max, that he had no insight regarding the independent steps he would need to take to be successful in getting a job. When I asked Max what he thought he needed to do, he replied, "Nothing really. I can just go there with Mom or Dad, have a chat with someone at the shop, and then see what happens next." When I raised the ideas of preparing a cover letter and resume, preparing for and attending interviews, and knowing how to respond to certain interview questions he seemed completely confused as to why he would be responsible for undertaking any of these steps. I think Max's example helps highlight the level of increased dependence—not independence—that seems to come with adolescence and autism.

Challenge to Risk Taking and Rebellion

It is sometimes argued that people with autism would make excellent policemen/women because they are so constantly mindful of what the rules and procedures are and exactly how they should be followed. Unfortunately, this stands in contrast to what is occurring for their typically developing peers who are fond of rebellion during their teenage years. You can imagine that, for a teenager with autism, it might be extremely unpopular and socially isolating to be the person who never takes risks, who often reminds others taking risks that they are doing something wrong, or who reports to authorities (e.g., tells their school principal) when someone breaks a rule.

Challenge to Socializing with Peer Groups

Given the known social difficulties of people with autism, it is not surprising that the adolescent years might be particularly anxiety provoking. While most typically developing teenagers are forming more solid relationships with their social group and moving away from their families, teenagers with autism are more likely to experience adolescence as a time of loneliness. By the teenage years, many people with autism are better able to understand that there are differences in social ability between them and their typically developing peers. They might know that they are not particularly good at keeping conversations going or finding a range of topics to discuss that their peers can relate to (e.g., most typically developing teenagers aren't interested in discussing various forms of public transportation). Social activities such as impromptu parties, late nights out with friends, and "hanging out" at a friend's house all day might involve challenges for any person with autism who seeks structure and routine, not spontaneity. Moreover, they might derive their sense of "fun" from exploring their own interest areas further rather than from hanging out and talking with friends.

One of my adolescent clients, Roland, has been struggling with these social differences for several years. He has come to understand that he is not skilled in keeping conversations going beyond his own interest areas in robotics and science fiction, and that he does not enjoy the lack of structure and rebellion that he often observes in his peers at parties or during breaks at school. That is, he has identified himself more as the "odd one out." Consequently, when he first came to see me he reported feeling lonely most of the time. Roland helps to highlight that for many people with autism there is a widening social gap between them and their peers, not a shrinking one, as is typically the case for adolescents who do not have autism.

What Are the Common Signs of Anxiety in Adolescents with Autism?

Anxiety Regarding Independent Living Skills

Teenagers with autism might feel less competent than their typically developing peers when it comes to living more independently and taking care of themselves. Tasks that require greater self-sufficiency and autonomy in adolescence including managing homework, planning and completing assignments, studying for exams, earning spending or pocket money, contributing to the general running of the family home, and taking responsibility for personal appearance might be particularly anxiety provoking. Indications that a teenager with autism is anxious in relation to these challenges might include:

- becoming easily overwhelmed by increased demands in school workloads;
- overreliance on parents to help complete school assignments;
- giving up on school tasks or procrastinating in completing them;
- refusing outright to complete learning tasks or to study for exams;
- an increase in seeking reassurance from parents regarding personal appearance;
- avoidance or lack of effort in caring for personal hygiene and appearance;
- becoming easily frustrated when parents remind her of personal hygiene or appearance issues;
- overreliance on parents to organize money earning opportunities out of fear that she cannot manage this herself; or
- fear and confusion regarding tasks such as researching casual job opportunities and preparing resources for job seeking.

Social Anxiety Regarding Risk-taking and Peer Interactions

Whether it is because they are not as rebellious or risk-taking as their peers or whether it is because they have more social interaction difficulties than their same age peers, many teenagers with autism are likely to experience a sense of social isolation. They might start to see themselves as "weird" compared with other kids their age. As a result, they are likely to experience significant levels of social anxiety regarding interacting with people their age. Signs of this social anxiety might include:

- reporting that they worry they will look silly or make a fool of themselves in front of their peers;
- reporting that they worry that others might laugh at them;
- reporting that they worry they might do or say something "wrong" or embarrass themselves;
- becoming easily overwhelmed during conversations with their peers and forgetting what they were going to ask or say;
- avoiding social contact with other people their age;
- declining invitations from their peers to go out and socialize;

- refusing to attend school;
- seeking repeated reassurance from parents regarding the appropriateness of the way they speak or the topics they talk about;
- referring to themselves as socially incompetent; e.g., "dumb," "weird," "loser," "loner"; or
- loss of confidence around or avoidance of the opposite sex.

Anxiety in Adults with Autism

What Are Some of the Key Characteristics of "Normal" Adult Development?

Developing Love and Intimacy in Relationships

By adulthood (particularly by our mid-twenties), we are focused on forming good relationships with others whether they are friendships or more intimate relationships. Adults without autism hone skills of listening to and supporting other people emotionally, committing to another person, making sacrifices for other people, sharing goals with other people, and remaining loyal to close friends and loved ones. Essentially, we are establishing the ability to show other people that we love them and that we need their love.

Developing a Sense of Contentment and Secure Self-esteem

As adults, we also aim to develop a sense of security or contentment with who we are. That is, we aim to establish good self-esteem. In adulthood, we tend to look back over our experiences, difficulties, achievements, and relationships with a sense of satisfaction regarding how they have contributed to developing our identities and helped us to make life choices accordingly.

How Does Autism Affect These Stages of Adult Development?

Challenge to Developing Love and Intimacy

Adults with autism certainly have and can show a capacity to love other people. However, their social and communication difficulties make it hard for them to experience "intimacy" or closeness to other adults in the way we might typically expect to see demonstrated or communicated. For adults with autism, displaying tenderness or finding ways to show friends that you are "thinking of them" and supportive of them might be difficult. At times, their attempts might seem robotic, awkward, lacking in intense emotion or passion. Moreover, their communication difficulties might make it particularly difficult for them to communicate with loved ones about their hopes, their emotions, their hurts, or their frustrations as is commonly discussed in most relationships among typically developing adult friends or couples.

Challenge to Developing Self-esteem

Adults with autism might be more likely than other adults to experience social difficulties, relationship difficulties, communication difficulties within their workplace, and difficulties independently managing their daily living tasks. Therefore, if they consider these difficulties as a part of "who they are" or their identity, then they might feel frustrated with themselves. In turn, they might have low self-esteem rather than a sense of satisfaction with their life and their achievements.

What Are the Common Signs of Anxiety in Adults with Autism?

Anxiety and Depression

Adults with autism might be more likely than other adults to negatively evaluate their ability to be intimate with others and to be successful within their home life, their work life, and other daily living tasks. Therefore, by adulthood, the link between anxiety and depression might be quite strong. It is important that we are aware of these following warning signs:

- reporting dissatisfaction with achievements;
- reporting frustration with oneself and disappointment in oneself;
- blaming oneself for any social or relationship difficulties;
- avoiding opportunities for social interaction;
- judging oneself as "not good enough";
- lacking energy and motivation to complete daily living tasks;
- seeking repeated reassurance from friends or loved ones regarding choices and decisions;

Table 3	Some Common Signs of Anxiety across Development in People with an ASD	
Stage of Development:	Childhood
Situations or activities causing anxiety	■ Rules/rule breaking ■ Winning and losing ■ Making mistakes ■ Joining in and turn taking ■ Making friends
Anxious thinking	■ "I don't understand what is happening in the classroom." ■ "I don't know what to expect." ■ "The rules must always be followed." ■ "If I lose, then that means I'm not the best or the smartest." ■ "If I make a mistake, then my work won't be perfect." ■ "What if the other children won't play the game the way I want to play it?" ■ "What if the other children don't want to play with me?"
Anxious behavior	■ Bossiness ■ Scripting play, e.g., "You do this and I'll do that." ■ Crying ■ Tantrums ■ Aggression ■ Self-injurious behavior ■ Increased repetitive play ■ Increased stereotyped language ■ Increased repetitive movements ■ Avoiding social play

Adolescence	Adulthood
■ Rules/rule breaking ■ Performing in front of peers ■ Talking to peers ■ Making friends ■ Study and workload ■ Personal appearance	■ Relationships ■ Family ■ Workplace or career achievement
■ "The rules cannot be broken." ■ "I might make a mistake or embarrass myself." ■ "What if others think I'm weird?" ■ "No one wants to be my friend because they think I'm a loser." ■ "I won't be able to get this work finished." ■ "I don't look as cool as the other kids." ■ "I might get teased."	■ "I have made a mess of my life." ■ "I hope I haven't said or done the wrong thing to…" ■ "My family might be embarrassed by me." ■ "I might make a mistake at work." ■ "I'm not good enough to do my job properly." ■ "Other people seem to achieve more than me." ■ "It's my fault if my partner is unhappy. I've probably done something wrong."
■ Frustration ■ Aggression ■ Overdependence on parents ■ Excessively seeking reassurance ■ Giving up on or refusing to complete school tasks ■ Procrastinating ■ Avoiding social contact with peers ■ School refusal ■ Degrading themselves, e.g., calling themselves "dumb," "weird," "a loser," "a loner"	■ Avoiding opportunities for social interaction ■ Lethargy ■ Lack of motivation to complete daily living tasks ■ Poor sleep habits ■ Crying ■ Seeking reassurance from friends or loved ones regarding choices and decisions ■ Lack of effort in personal appearance ■ Loss of appetite ■ Pacing or other repetitive behaviors ■ Using drugs or alcohol

- harboring thoughts of self-harm;
- worrying about one's workplace behavior and communication style; and
- worrying about being accepted or liked by others.

Anxiety in Children with High Functioning Autism or Asperger's Disorder

Children with high functioning autism and Asperger's disorder are, by definition, more verbal than children with ASD who are lower functioning. Consequently, the ways they express anxiety might involve articulating more worries or using language to describe feeling fearful or worried. Also, by definition, children with high functioning autism are less likely to have intellectual delay. Therefore, they are better able to identify that they have communication and social difficulties. They are more likely to be aware of differences between them and their same age peers. Many parents tell me that their children have asked them questions such as "Why don't the other children speak like me?", "Why is it that I can't seem to make friends like the others?", "Why don't other children like talking about the same things as me?" These comments show that children can be aware that something is different between them and their peers. High functioning children's awareness of the social and communication gaps between them and other children might lead to more socially oriented worries. Specifically, they might worry more about fitting in with their peers, making a fool of or embarrassing themselves in front of their peers, or their peers evaluating them or judging them negatively. Recent research supports the idea that high functioning children with autism tend to have predominantly social worries (e.g., White, Oswald, Ollendick & Scahill, 2009). On that basis, we might expect to see more evidence of low self-esteem in high functioning children. If left untreated, significant anxiety and low self-esteem might be precursors to depression.

Other common areas of worry for children with high functioning autism and Asperger's disorder can include:

- worries about making or keeping friends,
- worries about winning and losing,
- worries about making mistakes,
- worries about perfectionism, and

- worries about school performance or performing in front of others.

In general, all of the above areas of anxiety seem to relate to the children feeling comfortable with themselves or their abilities in comparison with their peers.

Anxiety in Children with High Support Needs

Children who are more significantly affected by autism (i.e., intellectually delayed) might find it harder to clearly describe when they feel worried and why. Usually the language and communication difficulties are more marked in these children, making it harder for them to express themselves and their emotions. Therefore, we might be more likely to observe anxiety in the *actions* of these children rather than in what they *say*. Examples might include:

- challenging behavior when presented with a task that they find overwhelming;
- avoidance of people, objects, or tasks that they fear or find overwhelming;
- repetitive or stereotyped language or behavior in order to self-soothe; and
- self-injurious behavior.

One of the most interesting clients I see, seventeen-year-old Collin, is significantly affected by autism. Whenever he is anxious or fearful he seems to display the same patterns of behavior including:

- challenging behavior by swearing loudly and repeatedly out of frustration;
- avoidance of conversation regarding what he fears and talking to himself to indicate his preference to avoid what he fears, for example, "We don't have to talk about that" or "It's okay, I don't have to _____ if I don't want to;"
- stereotyped self-talk to self-soothe and allow himself to calm down by repeating to himself, "It won't be long now. I'm doing a good job";
- sweating and repeatedly wiping his face with a handkerchief; or
- scratching at or picking at scabs on his arms and legs.

In Summary

- Many of the stages of development from childhood to adulthood are affected by autism.
- This impact of autism creates a range of challenges and difficulties that might cause anxiety.
- The signs of anxiety in individuals with autism differ across childhood, adolescence, and adulthood. There are some important key signs of anxiety to watch out for at each of these stages in development.
- Signs of anxiety can differ between people with high functioning autism and those with higher support needs.

4 | Anxiety in Families

Angela and Nathan, parents of Thomas, nine years old with high functioning autism

Seeking advice regarding Thomas's schooling options, Angela and Nathan came to see me in order to arrange a review assessment of Thomas's current functioning. They wanted updated information on his overall development in order to determine what kind of school setting might be best for him. In their opinion, he had outgrown his current special school. Indeed, they were worried about his challenging behavior within the classroom including task refusal and "meltdowns" when limits were placed on him. He was a bright child whom they believed was capable of completing third grade work. Yet he was in a class where the curriculum was set at approximately a first grade level. The school seemed to think that Thomas was not completing the work because he was incapable of it, i.e., that his level of functioning was lower than what Thomas's parents believed.

There were very few options for alternative school placements for Thomas. He could attend a separate, supported class within a local mainstream school or he could be fully included. However, to date, all of the schools that Angela and Nathan had approached regarding Thomas either refused to accept his enrollment or provided an excuse as to why their school might not be the appropriate placement for him. They said things like "We're too far out of your area," "We have too little experience in supporting children like Thomas," "Thomas's reported challenging behavior might make it hard for him to feel comfortable at this school." Naturally, the constant rejections from schools not only distressed Angela and Nathan but also made them question their strong beliefs about Thomas's capabilities.

His parents believed that it was time to fully integrate him. They were seeking an assessment to confirm whether or not their expectation was realistic. However, they were extremely worried about whether or not they were making the right decision. Indeed, in most of our early sessions together Angela would end up crying, explaining that she felt she was out of options and did not know what to do next or what was best for Thomas.

Once the assessment seemed to confirm that full-time inclusive placement was a reasonable expectation for Thomas, Angela and Nathan then began to worry about how best to transition Thomas into this environment. Of course, there were also worries about how to navigate the new "political" system within the next school in terms of which teachers to meet with, when to pass information about Thomas onto the school, what information to pass onto them, and how to strike a balance between pushing for Thomas's support needs and allowing the school to make its own independent decisions. Again, many sessions were spent with Angela ending up in tears with a sense of being overwhelmed about what decisions to make next.

Ian, father of Andrea, seven years old

Ian came to see me regarding concerns about Andrea's ability to cope in competitive social experiences, for example playing games or team sports with peers that involve winning and losing. He discussed feeling particularly worried about what happens whenever Andrea loses in a board game or during a sporting match. He described that she tantrums, spends the rest of the time at home sulking, refuses to talk to him or her mother, or at times either throws objects in her room or slams doors in the house out of frustration. He described that he was unable to reason with Andrea when she behaved this way.

Ian revealed that he felt highly anxious about Andrea's difficulties with winning and losing. For example, he stated, "My heart is in my mouth every time I pick her up from soccer practice. I'm always worried that she'll be in a bad mood because she has not played as well as the other members of her team." He recalled one incident wherein Andrea had walked off the field during a practice session to sulk because she had missed a goal.

Despite the difficulties with being competitive, Andrea seemed to have a small circle of friends at school. Teachers also seemed to report that Andrea was doing "okay" socially with her peers and joining in well in games on the playground. However, Ian indicated that he was unwill-

ing to allow Andrea to socialize out of school in case she ended up in a competitive situation with another child or group of children. Therefore, he would not allow Andrea to attend friends' birthday parties nor to participate in out-of-school play dates at this stage. Instead, Andrea's parents would arrange family activities over weekends or school holiday periods that Andrea could participate in without including her school friends. In other words, Ian was avoiding allowing Andrea to have social experiences outside of school in case her behavior became too competitive. He further reported that he had pulled Andrea out of soccer for the following season because of her tendency to become upset if the team lost or if she didn't score a goal.

Until now we have been exploring what anxiety is as well as how and why it might manifest in people with an ASD. However, the examples above highlight that anxiety also significantly affects the people immediately around the person with autism, especially the parents. In the example of Angela, there are a number of pressures and stressors that seem to burden her as she tries to make the best decisions regarding where to place her child for school. These stressors are common among almost all parents that I work with. In Ian's description, his own anxiety affects the decisions he makes concerning the limitations he placed on his child's social experiences and the avoidance of possible social "failures" for her. Perhaps the descriptions and information in this chapter might help parent readers recognize what the common stressors can be on them as well as when they might be modeling their own anxious behavior for their child. If parents can understand what triggers anxiety in themselves, then they'll be better prepared to implement the strategies discussed in the remainder of this book (Chapter 5 onward). As you read this chapter, be aware that practical solutions for dealing with these issues will be specifically addressed in Chapter 9.

Common Sources of Anxiety for Parents of Children with Autism

Across all of the developmental stages of children with an ASD, there are likely to be many sources of pressure and anxiety for parents. In general, I think that these sources of stress or anxiety fall into three broad areas outlined below.

Managing Challenging Behavior

In my years of experience in this field, it seems that coping with the challenging behavior of a child with an ASD can be the biggest source of stress and anxiety for parents. Parents seem to dread the possibility of a "meltdown" from a child because of the associated tension and multi-layered stress it brings: stress for the child who is frustrated, stress and sometimes embarrassment for the parent having to manage the child's behavior, and stress for the other family members (e.g., siblings) who observe the behavior regularly. Common examples of challenging behavior in people with an ASD include:

- *Those who have limited communication skills and cannot clearly explain what they want or when they need help and so scream or tantrum until the parent seems to pick the right option.* For example, a child who cannot express to a parent that he needs help fixing a broken toy is likely to cry or tantrum until the parent examines the toy and determines what is wrong and how to fix it.

- *Those who react to changes in their personal environment or routines or changes in the broader environment.* For example, a child who becomes very frustrated when a parent gets a haircut and appears somewhat different than usual.

- *Those who tantrum when they cannot access what they want.* The classic example we all think of is when children who are prevented from playing with their preferred toy or prevented from purchasing a new toy at a shop suddenly tantrum.

- *Those who are confused because they are unable to interpret or understand the subtleties of a social interaction.* For example, a person who does not understand that another's playful teasing is one way of being friendly might overreact with anger or distress.

- *Those who become challenging when an activity does not proceed as they had expected.* For example, a person who acts out when he is expecting to engage in an activity like going to the beach, but is unable to because the weather changes and prevents him from going.

■ *Those who become anxious and frustrated when they set unrealistic goals for themselves that they do not reach.* For example, a child who believes that he should get 100 percent of his spelling words correct on a test, despite having difficulties with written expression and spelling, and then runs out of the classroom when he discovers that he has made several mistakes.

In all of the above examples, it is typically an adult—usually a parent—who is required to help the child manage his emotions and behavior. Parents need to be skilled in using a range of responses for challenging behavior depending on why the behavior is occurring. The repertoire of possible responses might include distracting the person, ignoring the behavior, using discipline (e.g., time out), implementing a punishment (e.g., removing a privilege), or trying to rationalize/reason with the person. Being able to interpret why a child engages in challenging behavior and, therefore, which type of response to use in each situation is not a skill that we are born with. Parents have to work hard to understand the function of challenging behavior and the most effective ways to manage it across each of the situations described above. Clearly, this might be a source of stress, pressure, and anxiety for a parent. Many have described to me the instant tension, embarrassment, and fear they feel when their child engages in what is commonly described as a "meltdown." They might panic about trying to understand what it is that is causing the behavior and, therefore, how to respond. In a public place, the experience is almost unbearable for many parents who often report "giving in" in order to keep the child calm and prevent causing "a scene."

An empirically proven method to determine why a particular behavior is occurring is called a "functional behavior analysis" (FBA) (see the definition box). Specialists, such as psychologists or behavior therapists, are able to help parents complete an FBA regarding their child's "problem" behavior, including anxiety related behaviors. Alternatively, a school professional might be able to do this also. Understanding why a behavior occurs puts parents and professionals in a better position to address the cause of the anxiety and extinguish the problem behavior.

70 | Anxiety in Families

What Is Functional Behavior Analysis (FBA)?

Put simply, functional behavior analysis is a technique used to analyze or "work out" why a specific behavior is occurring. Usually, an FBA involves keeping a diary about what is happening before the behavior occurs (the antecedents), what exactly occurs when the person demonstrates the behavior, and what the results of the behavior are (the consequences). By keeping some written record or diary about the target behavior in this way, we are able to see whether there are any patterns. We might see whether there are common environments or triggers that lead to the behavior occurring. We might also see patterns in terms of what the person gains or gets from displaying the behavior. For example, we might see that whenever a child is presented with a writing task, he has a "meltdown" and is then usually sent out of the classroom. In this example, the child is getting what he wants—he "gains" an opportunity to avoid the task. Therefore, we might conclude that the purpose or "function" of the challenging behavior (meltdown) is to avoid the writing task.

Making Decisions

The case example of Angela and Nathan above helps emphasize another common source of stress that adults, particularly parents, experience in supporting a person with an ASD: making decisions. For all of us, life is full of turning points and times when we have to make important decisions by carefully considering both short- and long-term consequences. For adults supporting people with autism, especially parents, decision making seems to happen more frequently because of the special needs of their children. Things that others might assume or take for granted cannot be assumed for someone with autism. For example, on a very simple level, we might assume that a child would like to go to the park to play and run around, therefore making the decision to take him there an easy one. But for a child with autism, we might need to consider other factors such as which route to take to go to the park, whether there will there be too much noise at the park, whether the child will try to dominate some of the play equipment and have difficultly taking turns with the other children, or if the child will wander off because he observes some sticks or rocks that he decides to go off and collect as a part of a special or unusual interest. If we can see that a simple trip to the park might become a source of anxiety for parents, then imagine the kind of pressure that might be on adults regarding other, even more significant, decisions as outlined below:

What Type of Early Intervention Is Best for the Child?

Both professionals and parents can find this question very challenging. Knowing that early intervention is the best predictor for long term outcomes in people with autism, the choice as to which method to follow is a source of anxiety for many adults supporting people with autism. They fear that making the "wrong choice" will lead to poorer outcomes for their child's development of communication and social skills. Common questions include: Is intensive applied behavior analysis (ABA) more suitable for our child than Floortime™? How many hours of intervention are enough? Which service provider is the most suitable for our child and family? How are we going to afford the intervention? Will my child be able to speak after speech therapy begins? How will we measure whether or not the intervention is working? What if the intervention doesn't work? Should I put my child on a special diet?

Where Do I Get Information On...?

Nowadays, I have found that access to information on autism and how best to support people with it can be just as anxiety provoking and confusing as it can be helpful for both parents and professionals. Within the field, there is a mix of both evidence-based strategies and interventions as well as other more "questionable" or alternative approaches. As a professional or parent, how do you tell the difference and where do you access the right information to help you decide which is evidence-based and which is not? Is researching online enough? Do you speak to another professional? Do you attend a parent support group and ask other parents about their own personal experiences? Do you research scientific journals or attend international conferences? From my experience in the field, all of these sources seem to contain a mix of the helpful, the misleading, and even the unethical. For example, lately, the "University of Google" has become a significant source of information for parents. However, if you search the term "autism," I'm sure you will find that a mix of links appear—from large organizations at the forefront of research about autism to homeopathic remedies that promise a "cure" without any solid, scientifically-researched evidence to back them up. Often, parents trying to provide their children with the best opportunities to develop and reach their full potential are vulnerable to falling for strategies that are well marketed, even if what is suggested is basically useless. Professionals and parents often feel that they struggle to access information from reliable sources on "what to do when…." Unfortunately, there is no one universally supported autism handbook that provides a complete summary of everything about autism and how to best manage it, because each individual with autism is indeed that—an individual.

What School Setting is Best?

Angela's tears and worry for Thomas in the example above highlight the stress many parents suffer when choosing an appropriate school or setting for their child. The most common questions regarding schooling that I have had to help find answers to include:

- What school setting will be best for my child?
- Should I send him to school next year or hold him back at preschool another year?
- Is full-time inclusion with some support from a teacher's aide better than a supported classroom within a mainstream school?
- Will my child require the support of a special school and for how long?
- What if the children at a special school model more challenging behavior for my child?
- Is a public school or a private school better for my child?
- What if the school is not open to having a child with special needs?
- How do I explain my child's needs to the school?
- I don't want people to be prejudiced toward my child. Do I have to tell the school that my child has autism?
- How do I arrange for more support for my child at the school?
- How do I help my child make friends at his school?
- Does my child have to do the same amount of homework as the other children?
- Does my child *have* to participate in sporting events?
- Can I attend school fieldtrips with my child in case he doesn't cope well?

- Should I try to arrange for my child to attend school part-time then build up to full-time hours?
- Should I try to make regular times to meet with professionals at my child's school to monitor his progress or is that being too "pushy?"

As you might appreciate, there is no right or wrong answer to any of the questions above. Each individual with autism is an individual first and, therefore, each person has different education and support needs. However, for a parent or for a professional guiding the parent, the need to get the balance right can certainly be a source of anxiety, most often because of the unspoken questions that loom in the back of the mind: "What if I make the wrong decision and the child is unhappy there?" and "What if I make the wrong decision and the child misses out on a window of valuable learning time that he can't make up for?"

Adjusting Expectations

A third common source of stress for adults who support a child with an ASD is that of adjusting expectations. From the point of diagnosis, many parents experience anxiety trying to constantly adjust and readjust the expectations that they had or have for their child. It is hard for them to determine at each stage of their child's development what to expect of their child and what their child's potential might be. Consequently, parents find it difficult to determine whether or not to push their child to develop more skills based on their expectations. For example, parents might find that they significantly readjust their expectations for their child from what they had been around the time of the initial diagnosis to what they might need to be once the child has completed several years of early intervention. That is, often the child is capable of achieving more than the parent was first told to anticipate because of quality early intervention. Of course, this is a positive adjustment for parents to make; however, it can still involve much anxiety as plans they might have made based on recommendations at the time of the child's diagnosis might need to change suddenly (e.g., plans for school placement). The following story of the York family represents a good example of readjusting expectations and anxiety surrounding this process.

The Yorks, parents of Angus, five years old

When Angus was first diagnosed with autism at just over two years of age, it was unclear what type of schooling option might be most suitable for him in the long term. At the time, his development was defined as borderline to mildly delayed and so the family was told that supported education, such as a special autism class in a mainstream school or special school, might be the most appropriate setting for him. However, in the three years before Angus turned five and was ready to attend formal schooling, his family made incredible efforts to provide a range of quality interventions for him including behavior therapy, speech therapy, parenting support, and psychology services. When Angus was assessed at the end of the year, before he was ready to attend school, it was determined that his developmental level was more likely low average to average for his age and that an inclusive setting would be the most appropriate option for him.

Despite the very positive outcome for Angus, his parents now faced the dilemma of where to send him as they had planned around the original suggestion of a special autism class in a mainstream school. Angus's parents became highly anxious about this new decision. They arranged weekly meetings with me to help them ensure that all of their bases were covered in preparing Angus for mainstream schooling. Consultations also occurred between the preschool, myself, and the parents to try to set up more visual work systems for Angus so that he could become more independent in completing a string of activities without being "shadowed." His parents indicated that they felt extremely pressured while working toward the deadline of the first day of school, trying to ensure that Angus was set up to succeed there. School meetings were another source of anxiety, especially for Angus's mother. She understandably found it difficult to accept that Angus was not going to receive as much support as she had thought he might have needed and was naturally worried about how Angus would cope in a large classroom of thirty students having to essentially "fend for himself" much of the time.

Commonly, parents report some fear or worry regarding adjusting their expectations for their child as the child moves into adolescence. Specifically, given their child's communication and social skill challenges they worry about: Will he cope at high school? Will he finish high school? Will he be able to have a relationship with someone? Will he get married and have his own family? Will he be able to find and maintain employment and manage his own personal finances? Ultimately parents worry about the question: Will he be able to care for himself and live independently? Usually, a diagnosis of autism implies that these milestones in development might not come as naturally as parents originally predicted or expected for their child. Consequently, the parents will need to frequently adjust and readjust what they expect of their son or daughter and, therefore, what their answers will be to these questions. For example, the Lang family is currently experiencing stress and anxiety regarding what expectations to reasonably have for their teenaged son, Michael, once he completes high school in two years time.

The Langs, parents of Michael, sixteen years old

Plans have begun for Michael to transition into some work experience and retail programs to supplement his final years at high school so as to prepare him for life outside of the structured school environment. Michael's parents have begun to worry about what to expect for him once he leaves school and has to manage even basic employment. They are fearful that Michael might not cope outside of the structured high school system and they feel uncertain about how well they will be able to assist him, themselves. It is the lack of clarity at this point regarding what expectations to have of Michael once he leaves high school that exacerbates his parents' anxiety as they feel confused about how best to help him and what might happen to him in the full-time workforce.

Frequently, parents I work with seem to experience anxiety in constantly trying to adjust their expectations around the question, "Does he do this because he has autism or is this normal for this current stage in his development?" This seems to be an especially common question for parents of small children with autism seeking advice regarding challenging behavior. Parents often try to determine whether the oppositional behavior they observe in their young child is simply "normal" for the child's age or whether a different kind of management strategy is required because the child has autism. Depending on the answer to that question, they might need to adjust and readjust their expectations of the child and how they respond to the child accordingly.

All of the issues described above—challenging behavior, decision making, and shifting expectations—can cause anxiety in parents.

Some tips on how parents can manage their own anxiety are outlined in Chapter 9.

Do Anxious Children Come From Anxious Parents?

There is now a body of solid research to show that typically developing children who experience anxiety difficulties tend to come from families where parents experience anxiety and display anxious behavior (Drake & Kearney, 2008; Hudson & Rapee, 2004; van der Bruggen, Stams & Bögels, 2008). I am sure this finding makes sense to many parents and the professionals who work with them. Clearly, this occurs in part due to heredity, but we also know that children learn from watching their parents and imitating them from an early age. This occurs also for any anxious behavior that a parent might display. If parents model anxious behavior, then children—whether they have an ASD or not—are likely to pick up on the sense of anxiety or worry and behave in a similar way. There are six key ways that parents can unwittingly model anxious behavior for their child.

1. Questioning

Parents can model anxiety for their child by questioning whether or not the child feels comfortable in any given situation. Questions such as *Are you alright?*, *Do you want me to come with you?*, *Do you think you can manage _____?*, *Do you want me to check for you?*, *Do you think that's okay for you or are you a bit worried about it?* are all examples of questions that anxious parents might often ask. Obviously, parents ask these questions with the best of intentions. They have their child's best interests at heart. However, what the parent might not realize is that he might be indirectly undermining the child's confidence. Specifically, asking whether the child is okay or can manage something implies to the child the possibility that there might be some reason to worry or some reason that he might not be able to manage. Consequently, what the parent intends as a supportive question can actually serve to undermine the child's confidence and increase the child's anxiety. The following example may help to illustrate this point.

Usually I meet with a child individually (i.e., without his parents) after first meeting with the parents or the whole family. When it came time for me to meet Jack individually, I walked into the waiting room as I normally do, said hello and invited Jack to come with me for "some playtime and a chat." Jack got up and began to follow me. However, out of care and concern for Jack, his mother immediately asked, "Jack, are you alright? Are you okay to go with Dr. Chalfant on your own or do you want me to come with you?" At this option, Jack stopped, looked at me, looked at his mother, and then walked over to her and sat back on her lap. His mother then stated, "Yeah, I thought he'd be uncomfortable on his own. I think I'd better come in with him for a while." Of course, this was not a problem. Jack began the session with both me and his mother present and then after some "warm up" time, I suggested that Jack might be fine to continue with me alone and his mother went back to the waiting room.

The point to make here is that Jack seemed to question himself and change his behavior because of his mother's questioning of him. Again, it was clear that his mother asked these questions out of love and care; however, ultimately they also seemed to shake Jack's observed confidence in attending the session alone.

There are no hard and fast rules regarding exactly how many questions are too many and what amount is anxiety provoking vs. what amount is reasonable. However, if parents become more aware about the possible impact of the way they speak to their children then that is a positive start to reducing any anxiety.

2. Checking

Again, with good intentions, some anxious parents worry about their child's successful performance at school and check their child's work for errors. However, there is a fine line between checking over a child's spelling list for mistakes and insisting on looking over all completed work in case there are errors that need correction before homework is handed in. In life, we all need to learn from our own mistakes rather than be prevented from making them altogether. The importance of learning from our own mistakes applies to people with an ASD too. They need to learn from their own mistakes in order to learn to work independently.

Parents who can be slightly perfectionistic might pass on these traits to their children. Children with parents who seem to check or try to perfect work or activities the children have engaged in (e.g., homework, a sports skill, a social skill) might be prevented from feeling comfortable in attempting the work or activity without help. That is, they might begin to automatically call on the parent or another adult for assistance even though they might be quite capable of completing work independently.

Michael's parents worry about his literacy skills because of his communication difficulties and his language delay. Consequently, they take turns checking all of Michael's reading, writing, and spelling with him to ensure that his work is error-free. While Michael's parents are trying to help him develop better literacy skills and be supportive of him, Michael no longer feels comfortable attempting any literacy task (even those below his current reading and spelling levels) without an adult sitting alongside him to watch for errors. Michael has learned to rely on an adult to find and correct his errors. Therefore, he no longer feels confident working independently.

3. Safety Seeking or Overprotective Behavior

Parents of people with an ASD are the ones who most often witness their child's frustration and disappointments when situations do not evolve as the child might wish. They are the people with the most first-hand experience observing "meltdowns" when their child does not get what he wants. Sometimes, parents go to great lengths to prevent the child from becoming distressed and engaging in challenging behavior. These efforts are sometimes referred to as "safety seeking" or "overprotective" behaviors. They are behaviors that the parent might engage in to help the child feel safer or more comfortable and, therefore, to prevent him from experiencing any possible distress. Some examples of safety seeking behaviors are outlined below:

- Parents who knew that their child was anxious about arriving to appointments on time ensured that they took their child to school fifteen minutes early everyday to try to guarantee that the child would not become upset.
- Parents who knew that their child would become very upset whenever he lost a game would deliberately allow the child to win to avoid the possible tantrums that might occur.

- Parents who knew that their child hated handwriting because of his poor fine motor skills would either complete the work for the child or tell the child that he would ask the teacher if he could be exempt from writing tasks altogether.
- Parents who knew that their child became distressed using the toilet for a bowel movement because of difficulty wiping himself properly used to wait vigilantly by the bathroom door and complete the wiping for the child so as not to distress him.

Again, in each of the above examples, it is clear that the parents are concerned for their children and are trying to prevent further distress or frustration. However, anxious parents are more likely to go to great efforts to "safety seek." In turn, they prevent their children from learning the lesson that arriving late for school or losing a board game is not the end of the world; handwriting is difficult but I can improve slowly; or, over time, I might be able to learn how to wipe myself after I use the toilet even though it seems "yucky."

4. Avoidance

Some anxious parents choose to avoid situations that might cause distress for their child and, in turn, themselves. Unfortunately, what this falsely teaches the child is that it is safer to avoid an anxiety-provoking situation than it is to participate in it. There are several classic examples of avoidance that I see regularly in my own practice; i.e., parents who determine that it is better to prevent their child from participating in field days, school camping trips, or assemblies. They choose this option rather than allow their child to attend a part of the field day, camp, or assembly, or to take on a special job within them, e.g., become the time keeper for the swimming races. In these examples, the child is prevented from learning that he could possibly cope with the anxiety he experiences at one of these events. Rather, avoidance reinforces the child's and the parents' beliefs that such activities or events are not safe for the child. Again, detailed strategies to assist parents in dealing with their child's temptation to avoid anxiety-provoking activities are discussed in Chapters 5 and 8.

5. Reducing Independence

Anxious parents are more likely to complete activities with their child or for their child than allow the child to try it alone and experience a possible mistake, problem, or "failure." Again, such parents have loving intentions in trying to help their child; however, always trying to assist a child stifles his ability to become independent and reduces the child's confidence that he can accomplish a task on his own. A common example of this that I see in my work are the parents that believe that, because of their child's limited social skills, they need to accompany their child to all play dates, parties, and other social occasions. They do so even if there is already other adult supervision there. In this example, such parents might be indirectly teaching their child that he is unable to cope socially without the parent alongside him, in case something goes "wrong."

Again, there are no clear rules regarding when to take a step back from your child and when to allow his dependence upon you. However, perhaps one way for a parent to objectively evaluate whether to help his child or not could be based on whether the child has even the most basic skills necessary to engage in a task or situation alone, even if he makes some mistakes. For example, a child who has some ability to greet other children and participate (even passively) in a game with them might be best given only minimal assistance from his parent vs. a child who has no command of these skills whatsoever. Chapters 5 and 8 outline suggestions to help parents increase independence in their child.

6. Paying Too Much Attention to Non-brave Behavior

When children become anxious or worried, anxious parents are more likely than non-anxious parents to pay extra attention to this kind of behavior (Gar & Hudson, 2008; Gar, Hudson & Rapee, 2005). They may fret, or show distress or concern in front of the child if the child is upset instead of remaining calm or neutral—playing down the child's worries or distracting the child. For example, David reported to his mother that he was not picked to be first in his line at school. He told her that because of this he ran away from the classroom. David's mom instantly began to soothe him, put him on her lap, and cuddle him. She became upset at seeing his distress. Finally, she tried to comfort him by offering him a special treat, namely a new toy. Naturally, David's mom acted out of care for David; however, it is possible that a general lesson was modeled for David: non-brave or non-coping behavior (e.g., running away) is met with warm hugs and treats and lots of one-on-one attention. Therefore, David might be more likely to show similar lack of coping next time he is not picked to be first in the school line.

The above six ways in which anxious parents can model anxious behavior for their children with an ASD highlight that what they try to do out of care and love for their child can have unforeseeable negative consequences. In particular, parents who model any of the six responses discussed above might inadvertently be increasing their child's dependence and worry, and reducing their child's self-confidence.

Anxiety in Siblings

A recent Australian film, "The Black Balloon," depicted the life of a family with an adolescent with autism named "Charlie," seen mostly from the perspective of his typically developing sixteen-year-old brother named "Thomas." Examples of Charlie's impulsive and challenging behavior include spending hours amusing himself by banging a pot with a wooden spoon, having a tantrum in a supermarket, and running down the street wearing his underpants and a hat with mouse ears. Thomas is portrayed as experiencing immense anxiety and pressure in trying to live with and manage Charlie's challenging behavior. Thomas seems anxious about being seen with his brother for fear of being teased or bullied by his peers. He is also anxious about bringing his new girlfriend to the house in case his brother engages in any inappropriate behavior that might make her like Thomas less. Thomas is lacking in self-confidence and somewhat misunderstood by his parents, whom he feels do too much to support his brother and, consequently, less by way of spending time with him. Although I am not a movie critic, I believe that this film does an excellent job of portraying the mix of emotions and worries that a sibling of a person with autism can experience. Below are some of the key areas to be mindful of for siblings.

Taking On Too Much Responsibility

It is not unusual for siblings of people with autism to take it upon themselves to carry more responsibility in the family. They might do this in order to assist parents in coping with managing and supporting the family member with special needs. At times, this extra responsibility can mean that siblings "grow up" in a short period of time compared to their peers. They may become involved in their brother or sister's intervention or therapy or in assisting in the completion of self-care routines at home. In the film described above, Charlie and Thomas's mother is pregnant with the family's third child. Consequently, Thomas takes on extra responsibilities for managing some of his brother's daily living activities including organizing meals and assisting in bathing him. You can imagine that most teenagers might prefer to be spending time out of the home with peers and pursuing their own interests. Therefore, it seems like a significant sacrifice to make at a young age to take on more of a "parenting" role in the household. Thomas's experience is not uncommon for many siblings regardless of the level of functioning of the person with autism (in the film, Charlie is clearly someone with very high support needs).

I began working with a delightful young girl named Valerie for her anxiety difficulties when she was only seven years old but she seemed more like a fourteen-year-old. She demonstrated a strong sense of responsibility for her younger brother and, indeed, her whole family. She seemed to have taken it upon herself to be directly involved in caring for her younger brother, Lachlan, who has autism. Although Lachlan is high functioning, Valerie still seemed to feel responsible for making sure that he followed the household routines and completed tasks, like homework. She also spent time ensuring that he practiced social skills when they were in public places such as the park.

Excessive Worry about Other Family Members

Valerie's care for her brother was beautiful to observe. However, the excessive worry she had concerning her brother's development and the happiness of other family members was causing her significant difficulty. She was not eating or sleeping well. She lost confidence in her own ability to make friends and to complete school work. She was falling behind in key learning areas such as reading and written expression. When I first met Valerie she said that she worried on a daily basis about her brother and whether or not he would ever make "good friends." She also reported daily worries regarding her parents and whether or not they would have enough money to be able to afford Lachlan's interventions as well as activities like movies and vacations. She felt guilty that she was attending a private school, which she knew cost more money than if she attended the local public school. She worried about the parents' small business and how viable it was when her mother had to spend so much time taking her brother to and from appointments with various healthcare professionals. Clearly, all of Valerie's worries were quite "adult" for a child just seven years of age. It is important to be aware of any excessive (e.g., daily) worry in siblings of people with autism so that they do not feel more pressure than what is reasonable to expect of other children their age. Chapter 9 contains some useful strategies to help prevent and/or manage anxiety in siblings.

Social Anxiety

Despite the increasing community awareness and growing support for people with autism, it does still seem that there is stigma attached to any individual with this diagnosis. Therefore, it is not surprising that siblings of people with autism are also aware of this stigma. Consequently, they might feel somewhat socially anxious because of it. In sibling support groups it is common to hear children identify feeling self-conscious or worried about what their friends or classmates think of them. They report feeling embarrassed to invite friends over to the house in case their brother or sister behaves in a way that might bother their friends. For example, they might worry about their sibling interrupting their play or engaging in some kind of stereotyped or repetitive behavior that their friends might see as "weird." Some siblings report feeling worried that their peers will think that there is something "wrong" with them. That is, they worry that their peers think that each member of the family might have features of autism too. Some siblings worry about their peers making fun of their brother or sister and, in turn, humiliating them. As noted above, in "The Black Balloon," Thomas seemed to experience social anxiety regarding how his school peers would react to him because of his brother. Indeed, in some instances, the less sensitive students at Thomas's school did tease him by mocking his brother Charlie and pretending to imitate Charlie's stereotyped behaviors. This served to make Thomas more anxious about being seen with or near his brother. He seemed to worry that by associating with Charlie, his peers might think he was "weird" too.

Loss of Confidence or Low Self-esteem

Although not deliberately planned, usually the child with autism demands and is given more attention and support than the sibling without autism. From early intervention to transitioning to supported employment, it is common for the person with autism to require more support from parents and professionals than his typically developing sibling. Naturally, extra support requires extra care, time, and attention. However, from a sibling's perspective, the reduced attention and time away from him can make him feel like he is viewed as less important or less special. Consequently, the sibling might lose self-confidence and self-esteem. An example of loss of confidence can be seen in Catherine's story below.

Trent's sister, Catherine, is four years older than he. She has been involved in Trent's intervention and appointments with healthcare professionals from approximately six years of age, at times being used as a pseudo-tutor for him to help teach appropriate social and communication skills by practicing therapy activities and role plays with Trent. Catherine has reported that she finds it frustrating at times that Trent seems to get "all of the attention" at home from their parents. Catherine also tends to act somewhat socially shy and reserved. Her mother reported that Catherine often describes negative thoughts about herself such as, "I'm not good enough. The other girls at school look better than me. I'll never be really good at anything."

Catherine's negative self-talk is not a direct result of something that Trent or her parents have done. However, it might seem reasonable to suggest that the likely imbalance in support or attention that Catherine indicates she observes in the family contributes to her limited self-image. Therefore, of late, we have been spending more time working with Trent's parents on ways to spend more time with Catherine.

(Some of these strategies are outlined in Chapter 9.) We have also been developing strategies for Catherine's parents and her high school teachers to help boost Catherine's self-confidence.

It is important that anxiety difficulties in the family of a person with autism do not go unchecked and unsupported. In Chapter 9 we'll look closely at strategies for anxious family members (parents and siblings) to adopt. The strategies are designed to help reduce anxiety and boost self-confidence and self-esteem in family members.

In Summary

- Anxiety can be a common experience for both the parents and the siblings of an individual with autism.
- Parents can experience anxiety from a range of stressors including managing challenging behavior, making decisions about their child's intervention or schooling, and adjusting their expectations regarding what their child's full potential might be.
- Parents who already have traits of anxiety are more likely to have anxious children not only because they've potentially genetically passed it down but because they might model anxious behavior in front of their child.
- Although anxious parents have their child's best interests at heart, they might be more likely to reduce confidence and increase anxiety in their child. They can do this by:
  - giving excessive reassurance,
  - engaging in checking and safety seeking behaviors,
  - avoiding situations that make their child anxious, and
  - fostering too much dependence on them.
- Siblings of people with autism can experience anxiety from four key sources:
  - taking on too much responsibility within the family,
  - excessive worry regarding their family's welfare,
  - social anxiety, and
  - low self-confidence and self-esteem.
- It is important that possible anxiety difficulties in the family of a person with autism be closely monitored and addressed.

Part II

Indirect Treatments for Anxiety

5 | Treating Anxiety: Indirect Treatments for Use by Parents

Andrew and the Boyce Family

Currently, seven-year-old Andrew's anxiety manifests in his eating habits. He refuses to eat any food that is prepared by anyone other than his own mother. If asked to eat food prepared or touched by someone else, he becomes distressed and his behavior becomes challenging including having long-lasting tantrums.

Andrew will repeatedly ask before meals who has prepared his food, even if he knows that his mother has prepared it. When his mother refuses to answer him, Andrew again becomes distressed and challenging. Finally, his mother usually responds to him or reassures him. She reported that on a few occasions, when she has more resolve, she has been able to ignore Andrew's repeated questions. Eventually, he has eaten on these occasions. However, in general, Andrew's mother oscillates between trying to resist his questioning and responding to him when he is worried about food preparation.

Understandably, Andrew's resistance to eating food prepared by others makes life very challenging for the Boyce family. His mother might become exhausted and frustrated by being the only one to be able to prepare food in the home rather than share the load with others, like Andrew's father. Moreover, Andrew's parents have begun to argue over how best to manage his behavior. His father seems more inclined to want to set limits whereas his mother seems more inclined to try to rationalize with Andrew rather than "stress him out" too much. They have sought help to address Andrew's anxiety regarding eating because they do not know what approach is best to adopt. That is, do they refuse Andrew's control *regarding food preparation and "wait him out" with the tantrums that might follow, or do they avoid the distress and tantrums by complying with his eating preferences?*

The Anxiety Dilemma

In the example of Andrew above, it is clear that his parents face a dilemma over how best to manage his anxiety:

Option 1:

Do they allow Andrew to control how food is prepared at home and who prepares it so that they can avoid his experiencing distress and frustration? This option involves much interruption to the family's day-to-day functioning. For example, Andrew's mother is the only one "allowed" to prepare meals for him and this prevents the family from eating out at restaurants. Also, who will prepare Andrew's school lunches every day? What if Andrew's mother cannot be available all the time to organize his meals and food requirements? What can Andrew eat if he is to spend time at a friend's house? What happens if the family visits other people and food is prepared? What will the family do about Andrew's food and meal requirements if they go away on a vacation?

Option 2:

Do they gradually try to expose Andrew to food prepared by other people? This option might involve fewer demands on Andrew's mother, as the one who has had to spend time and energy planning and preparing his meals. However, this option is likely to involve some significant distress for Andrew, at least initially. His anxiety is likely to increase if he knows that someone other than his mother has prepared food for him. Also, this option might involve more challenging behavior from Andrew and, therefore, some distress for the family in trying to calm Andrew down and manage the behavior.

While both options involve difficulties for the family, in general it might be better for Andrew to learn to experience some anxiety and cope rather than avoid it altogether. In Chapter 4, the ways that parents might reinforce or increase a child's anxiety were outlined. By allowing anxious children to engage in "safety seeking" behavior we can perpetuate a child's anxiety. For Andrew, he is allowed to do this every time his mother agrees to be the only one to prepare food for him because it continues to make him feel "safe."

In this chapter, the anxiety dilemma for parents will be explored in more detail. A number of strategies that parents can use to help manage anxious behavior at home will also be outlined. These are not part of direct anxiety treatment programs (like the treatments and programs discussed in Chapters 7, 8, and 9). Rather, these strategies address the way parents engage with their anxious child and what techniques to use to increase the child's resilience and self-confidence. A child who is more self-confident is less likely to experience anxiety. Therefore, I call these parenting strategies "indirect" treatments because reductions in anxiety seem to happen indirectly as a result of changes in the child's confidence and sense of security. The strategies do not target the feared object or activity head on as with the strategies to be discussed in Chapters 7–9.

Encourage Bravery or Permit Avoidance?

As noted in the example of Andrew above, the Boyce parents are faced with a dilemma: Do they allow Andrew to have control of who cooks his meals and prepares his food or do they try to encourage Andrew to experience food prepared by someone other than his mother? Essentially, the dilemma faced by Andrew's parents reflects a broader issue that most parents of anxious children with autism will face: Do we encourage our children to face their fears or do we allow them to avoid what they are fearful of? Time and time again parents who come to me for assistance in managing their anxious child with autism will ultimately want an answer to the dilemma of whether to reinforce bravery or permit avoidance. Table 4 shows ten common examples from my own clients regarding the broad dilemma of encouraging bravery vs. permitting avoidance. It is likely that some of these are issues or questions you have faced or still face with your own child.

From Table 4 on the next page, you can see that although the topic area might be different, essentially the dilemma remains the same. So...what is the answer? Is it better to encourage bravery or to permit avoidance? Clearly, both options have their advantages and

Table 4	Common Anxiety Dilemmas for Parents	
Issue/ topic	**Encouraging bravery?**	**Permitting avoidance?**
Auditory stimulation (e.g., loud sounds)	Do I try to gradually desensitize my child to the sounds he is afraid of?	Do I avoid taking my child near any loud noises in case he becomes upset?
Homework	Do I break homework tasks down into small steps for my child to learn to complete?	Do I explain to my child's teacher that my child finds homework completion too stressful and she will only be able to complete tasks within the classroom?
Animals (e.g., dogs)	Do I try to make my child spend more time with dogs so she learns she can be safe?	Do I take my child to a different park where no dogs are allowed so as to avoid my child becoming distressed or interrupting her chance to play with other children?
Foods (e.g., taste aversion to meat sauce)	Do I try to gradually desensitize my child to the taste of Bolognese sauce?	Do I avoid giving meat sauces to my child because she cannot seem to tolerate them?
Play dates	Do I try to arrange play dates for my child so that she can learn to socialize more?	Do I avoid organizing play dates for my child because she has social difficulties and finds it stressful when play does not go according to her terms?
Winning and losing	Do I try to teach my child to cope with losing by playing games that she might lose?	Do I avoid games where my child might lose and become distressed?
School fieldtrips	Do I send my child on school fieldtrips?	Do I keep my child home from school fieldtrips that are not a part of the regular school routine and might confuse and cause distress for my child?

Making mistakes/ perfectionism	Do I teach my child coping strategies and that it's okay to make mistakes?	Do I allow my child to check her work repeatedly or get me to check it in order to prevent her from handing in imperfect work so that she doesn't become disappointed with herself?
Compulsive behaviors (e.g., shutting doors in the house)	Do I prevent my child from shutting all the windows and doors in the house every night?	Do I allow my child to shut all the windows and doors in the house each night because she feels more secure and can relax?
Changes in routine	Do I try to introduce more changes into my child's routine so that she learns to cope with change?	Do I try to avoid changes to my child's routines so that she does not become distressed or confused?

disadvantages. Perhaps the best way to answer this dilemma is to look at the likely outcomes of encouraging bravery vs. those of permitting avoidance and then decide which are better.

Encouraging Bravery

Encouraging bravery is likely to result in your child becoming distressed or anxious, at least in the short term. For example, if we encourage an anxious child who is fearful of certain sounds to listen to even a moment of that sound, then she is likely to experience distress or anxiety in doing so. However, we know from reviewing scientific research over the years (e.g., Tryon, 2005) that if an anxious person regularly experiences the object of her anxiety, her initial fear response will eventually shift to one of coping. Basically, the more we are exposed to objects or situations that might make us feel anxious, but are otherwise safe, the more likely we are to eventually learn that we can cope in those situations. Consider the example of my client, Benjamin, and his fear of dogs.

Benjamin was afraid of dogs and avoided them at all cost. He would seek support from a parent and try to run away or hide if he saw a dog. If there was a dog on television, he would try to change the channel. He also became upset if dogs were discussed in conversation. Benjamin believed that dogs were unsafe. He found their sudden movements frightening, believing that they might try to chase him and then eventually bite him.

Benjamin's parents chose the option of encouraging bravery. They discussed with Benjamin that they thought it best that he learn how to "boss away" his worries about dogs. They explained to him how his worries were being too bossy by stopping him from doing things like watching dogs on TV or remaining at the park when a dog was there. They told him they would help him become "the boss" over his worries so he could eventually control them. Benjamin's parents decided to prevent him from changing the TV channel when he saw a dog. They also began to discuss dogs more frequently at home. His parents were trying to teach him to cope with the idea of dogs rather than avoid dogs altogether.

Benjamin's parents found that when they first tried to prevent him from changing the TV channel he became extremely distressed and challenging by tantruming or throwing the remote control. However, they persisted. Although it took a long time (approximately one month), Benjamin was eventually able to remain in the room and watch a program about dogs or discuss dogs in conversation without becoming too distressed. Given Benjamin's shift to braver behavior, the family then began planning ways for Benjamin to have more "live" exposure to dogs. For example, they organized visits to the local pet shop and dog grooming service.

The example above highlights two points. First, even though Benjamin understood and accepted the idea of learning to "control his bossy worries," the family experienced short term difficulties in trying to encourage or push Benjamin to face his fears. Encouraging bravery is usually associated with initial increases in challenging behavior. Second, with persistence, the family was able to shift Benjamin's initial fear response to one where he could tolerate aspects of the object he feared. That is, in the longer term, they experienced success. However, the family had to be prepared to get past the short term difficulties in order to see the long term improvements in Benjamin's behavior and anxiety, and that isn't always easy to do.

Permitting Avoidance

By permitting avoidance, children are less likely to become distressed or anxious in the short term. For example, if we avoid particular sounds that cause anxiety for a child, then the child is less likely to have the opportunity to feel anxious or distressed. In a way, we are "saving" them from having to experience that distress. However, it is somewhat of a universal truth that, if an anxious person regularly avoids the object of her anxiety, then her anxiety level will ultimately increase—not decrease. This is because she will have fewer and fewer opportunities to see that she might cope in the presence of the object she fears. Basically, the less we are exposed to objects or situations that might make us feel anxious—but are otherwise safe—the less we are able to learn that those situations might be tolerable and the more likely we are to feel even more anxious the next time we do happen to face the fear. Consider the example of another of my clients, Jack, and his fear of losing.

Jack avoided playing games where he felt he might come off second best or worse. He would choose to play board games only with people he thought he could best. He would also change the rules of a team game (e.g., tag or soccer) midway if he felt that he was going to lose. At home, he would only play games with his parents if he was certain he could win. If he lost a game, he would become very frustrated and tantrum. Jack believed that winning was an indication that he was the "best." He did not like losing because he believed it meant that he lacked skills and was not as "smart" as the other people playing with him.

Jack's parents generally chose the option of permitting avoidance. For example, they would only ask to play games with Jack where they knew he would be able to win and, therefore, they could avoid his challenging behavior. They also allowed Jack to select friends for play dates according to whom he felt most comfortable with and, therefore, whom he felt would most accept him changing game rules or dominating the play. Jack's parents were trying to prevent Jack from feeling anxious or distressed about himself and his skills. Out of love and care for him, they were trying to protect Jack from experiencing low self-esteem or feeling that he was not as "smart" as other people. They wanted Jack to feel confident. Consequently, Jack's parents had few difficulties managing anxious behavior because they arranged Jack's play and games with him in such a way that he did not have an opportunity to become anxious. However, Jack's parents did notice that, over time, when Jack did play with a child at school who beat him in a game, his reactions were becoming more and more extreme. Specifically, after one incident at Jack's school in which he lost a handball game, the school called Jack's parents regarding a possible suspension because he had hit and injured another child out of frustration when he lost. In other words, over the long term, it seemed that despite his parents' efforts, Jack was actually displaying more anxiety when faced with the possibility of losing.

Jack's case highlights two important points. First, the family experienced short term relief in trying to avoid situations where Jack felt anxious. Simply, there were fewer opportunities for challenging behavior because Jack was able to win more frequently. Second, in the longer term, the family observed that, although Jack might experience anxiety less frequently (because he was losing less frequently), his anxiety level seemed to be increasing. When he was faced with a situation where he might lose, his reactions were becoming more extreme. Therefore, in the longer term, the family experienced greater problems.

Short Term Pain; Long Term Gain

Perhaps the best way to answer the dilemma of encouraging bravery or permitting avoidance is with the common slogan "short term pain, long term gain." Essentially, research and years of clinical experience have shown that it is better to encourage bravery in anxious children rather than to permit avoidance, even though doing so might lead to initial difficulties such as challenging behavior or distress. In the longer term, there are likely to be better outcomes for an anxious child who has been encouraged to face her fears and taught bravery than for an anxious child who has been allowed to avoid a feared object or situation.

What are the outcomes? One benefits of encouraging bravery is that the child is more likely to develop better coping skills. Therefore, she is likely to experience less anxiety in the longer term the more she is encouraged to be brave and face her fears.

A second benefit of encouraging bravery is that the child is more likely to develop independence. By encouraging bravery, you are also encouraging the child to learn to cope more independently. In Benjamin's case, he ultimately was able to stay in the room and leave the TV channel on or partake in conversation when the subject of dogs was discussed. Benjamin was learning to cope independently of his parents because he had to rely on himself to stay calm and remain in the situation rather than rely on his parents.

A third benefit of encouraging bravery is that the child is more likely to develop self-confidence and positive self-esteem. By increasing someone's coping skills and independence, we are helping her to develop more confidence in herself and stronger beliefs about her ability to face challenges. Consequently, she is more likely to feel positive about herself and less insecure or unsure.

Avoidance Increases Anxiety in Your Child

As was discussed in Chapter 4, it is very important that we do not indirectly increase a child's anxiety by avoiding what she fears, even though we love our child and usually have the best intentions in doing so. By avoiding the objects or situations that an anxious child with autism might fear, we are essentially preventing her from learning that she might actually be able to cope.

Going back to the ten common anxiety dilemmas that parents often discuss with me (Table 4), we might now see that it is better in the longer term to take the option of encouraging bravery than it is to permit avoidance.

To illustrate, total avoidance of sensory fears in children with autism will most likely serve to increase their anxiety toward these stimuli in the longer term. That is, the more we prevent children from hearing certain loud noises, the more likely they are to experience extreme distress the next time they happen to hear a sudden loud noise. Avoidance makes them less and less used to the stimulus and, therefore, less and less practiced in how to cope.

Similarly, the more we avoid sending our children on school fieldtrips because it might involve changing their routine and confusing them, the more likely they are to feel unable to cope when they do eventually attend a fieldtrip.

Further, the more we avoid particular animals that a child fears, the less practice the child has at coping with seeing the animal. The less ability she has to learn that the animal might actually be okay or safe—not as scary as she thinks.

And finally, the more we try to ensure that our routines do not change so as not to distress an anxious child with autism, the less able she will be to manage when there is a change. She will have had no practice in such an experience and feel less prepared and less able to cope.

Ultimately, if you want to help reduce anxiety in your child, then you need to be prepared to experience short term challenges in her behavior. You will need to allow your child to make mistakes. You will also need to allow your child to experience anxiety so that she can learn that the object she fears is perhaps not actually as bad as she believes it to be.

Strategies for Parenting an Anxious Child with an ASD

Given that encouraging bravery seems to be the better of the two options in the parent anxiety dilemma, what are the specific techniques and strategies that a parent can use to help encourage bravery in his or her child? The following are eleven strategies or "indirect treatments" to help parents reduce their child's anxiety and increase the child's coping, independence, and self-confidence. There are also some examples of how you might apply each strategy. However, these are merely suggestions. After reading them, you will probably be able to generate a more personalized list of techniques and examples for use in your own family. Depending on the age of your child and her level of support needs, you can explain to her what you are doing so that she knows to try to display brave behavior because she has your support and attention in doing so.

1. Praise Brave Behavior

As discussed in Chapter 4, sometimes we can allocate too much attention to anxious behavior. For example, we might spend time comforting people when they seem anxious. However, when they appear confident or able to cope, we tend to leave well enough alone, believing that they don't need extra attention. Actually, it is the reverse that is required. Put simply, we need to spend more time giving attention to brave or confident behavior and less time giving attention to fearful or anxious behavior.

One way to show that we are paying attention to brave behavior is by deliberately making an effort to find opportunities to praise a person for her bravery. Below are some examples. Keep in mind that you don't always need to use the word "brave." Depending on your child's age or vocabulary level, she might respond better to words like "confident," "independent," or "self-assured."

- "Wow, look how confident you were going over to that child and saying hello without my help!"
- "I am so proud of you for being so independent and doing your homework on your own."
- "Congratulations! You were so brave then when I told you that there would be a new visitor in your class today. You didn't look worried at all."
- "I can see that you are trying hard to walk on the path without being bothered by that dog over there. That is so brave of you!"
- "You let your brother have a turn at winning a point. It is amazing to see how brave you are trying to be."

For people with higher support needs, simpler statements might work better, for example:

- "Give me a high-five for being so brave!"
- "Awesome job staying calm."

Alternatively, positive behavior might also be used, for example, giving a reward (e.g., time with a preferred object or toy) as soon as you observe the child coping or staying calm.

You can see from the examples above that when praising brave behavior it is very important to use specific labels. It is vital to highlight key words or phrases like brave, independent, confident, doing it on your own, and giving it a try. Praising children for bravery helps them understand *exactly* what it is about their coping behavior that you like. Therefore, they are more likely to try to display it again. If you are the parent of an anxious child with autism, I recommend that you write up your own list of phrases or praising statements that really emphasize where you see bravery and confidence in your child. Then refer to the list as often as possible—several times each day. From the examples above you can also see that you do not need to wait for your child to conquer a death defying act in order to praise them for bravery. In fact, if you start by finding small examples of confidence and bravery then you'll probably find that you are able to praise them more often rather than if you are waiting for something "big" to happen.

2. Pay Close Attention to Brave Behavior and Independence

Beyond praise, we can allocate time and focus on brave and independent behavior in ways that really show someone we are paying close attention to her. This applies especially to a person with an ASD because we are positively reinforcing her behavior. In praising bravery, the focus is on verbal responses because we are using language to convey our delight or pleasure. However, we can also allocate attention and focus using lots of nonverbal behaviors including smiles, affection, high-fives, fist bumps, sitting alongside her and watching her eagerly, giving a concrete reward like a sticker or small toy, and engaging in silly or over-the-top behavior like dancing on the spot or doing a handstand in the kitchen out of celebration of her bravery. You know what makes your child happy, so use your own best judgment. Below are some ideas to get you started that can be applied to individuals with both high and low support needs:

- Walking over to your child when she is trying something new (e.g., a new food) and then giving her a big smile and/or cuddle as you tell her how proud of her you are for being brave and tasting something new.
- Stating something like "I noticed that you just chose your book for reading practice on your own, without my help. I'd love to sit beside you and listen to you read because I can see how confidently you are getting ready and I love to watch you when you are being confident."
- Doing a silly dance when you see that your child has coped with a change in her routine and perhaps even making up a playful song about it.
- Jumping in the shower or the pool with your clothes on when you see that your child has made a mistake with her homework without trying to correct it or re-do it until it is "perfect." (This kind of behavior might seem a bit over the top; however, parents I work with have actually done it and found it to be very effective).
- Giving your child a small treat or reward when she has been brave by reducing one of her compulsive or rigid behaviors. For example, allowing her to stay up ten minutes longer before bed or playing her favorite game with you

when she has allowed you to move one of her toy cars or
trains in the lines they repeatedly make on the floor.

For both verbal attention (e.g., praise) and nonverbal attention
(e.g., affection, time together, over-the-top behavior), it is critical that
you always respond **immediately** to your child. That is, you must
respond as soon as you notice her bravery or confidence. All children,
whether or not they have an ASD, benefit from instantaneous positive
reinforcement for their brave behavior rather than a response that
comes later in the day. Delayed responses make it harder for children
to see that your positivity is the direct result of something they have
done. For example, please *avoid* rewards and phrases such as "Because
you were so brave trying that new vegetable on your plate at lunch,
we'll go to the shop tonight and get you an ice cream cone as a special
treat." In this example, the reward of going out for an ice cream cone
comes too late after the actual brave act.

3. Set Goals

Often people become easily overwhelmed when they are anxious,
thinking that their fears are insurmountable. When we are trying to
conquer fears or worries it is always best to break the worry down into
smaller, more realistic and achievable steps. We are better off setting
smaller goals that we can work on one step at a time. Then, once we
have conquered a smaller goal, we feel more confident and less overwhelmed moving to a more challenging task. Even on a simple level,
setting goals can be done with people as young as approximately four
years of age. Depending on the age and level of support needs of your
child, you can sit down with her and talk her through the idea of setting
goals so that you work as a team with her in trying to conquer her fears.
Where possible, it is best that your child understands ahead of time
what the planned goals or steps are and how you'll help her achieve
those steps. Below are examples of how you might break down a worry
about dogs and a worry about being late into some smaller goals or
steps to be conquered one at a time:

Goal Breakdown for Overcoming a Fear of Dogs
- Goal/Step 1: Listen to someone read a book about dogs aloud.
- Goal/Step 2: Look at still pictures of dogs on the Internet.

- Goal/Step 3: Watch video footage of dogs on the Internet.
- Goal/Step 4: Stand outside the pet shop and look at dogs through the window.
- Goal/Step 5: Visit a friend or relative who has a dog and watch the dog play outside (while standing inside).
- Goal/Step 6: Stand outside and watch a dog while it is on a leash.
- Goal/Step 7: Pat a dog on a leash.
- Goal/Step 8: Play "catch" with a friend or relative's dog briefly for two minutes (with supervision or support from an adult).
- Goal/ Step 9: Play with a friend or relative's dog for ten minutes.

Goal Breakdown for Overcoming a Fear of Being Late

- Goal/Step 1: Accept the teacher's choice to start reading groups five minutes later than the usual time.
- Goal/Step 2: Accept Mom's/Dad's choice to turn the television on five minutes later than the usual time.
- Goal/Step 3: Walk in with Mom/Dad to swimming class five minutes late.
- Goal/Step 4: Walk in with Mom/Dad to swimming class ten minutes late.
- Goal/Step 5: Walk into swimming class, alone, five minutes late.
- Goal/Step 6: Walk into swimming class, alone, ten minutes late.
- Goal/Step 7: Be ten minutes late for school with Mom/Dad to explain why to the teacher.
- Goal/Step 8: Be twenty minutes late for school with Mom/Dad to explain why to the teacher.
- Goal/ Step 9: Be ten minutes late for school and, alone, explain why to the teacher.

It is important that we set realistic goals and start with the goal or step that seems most manageable or easiest to achieve. Again, we want to set the individual up to succeed, so going straight to Step 9 on the list above would not lead to success. The more we practice each step or work towards each goal, the more likely we are to feel comfortable doing it.

You can make goal-setting an engaging activity for your child by including her in the preparation of the steps or goals. For example, you could prepare a chart or stepladder of goals on the computer with your child or make one as a craft activity together.

4. Proportional Rewards

For each of the steps or goals that are set and conquered, it is vital that there is a reward. Depending on the age and level of support needs of the person, you can tell her ahead of time what rewards you will give and what she is "working towards." However, in general, it is a good idea to "deliberately plan" to surprise the person with the reward whenever you notice her bravery so that, from her perspective, the reward seems more spontaneous and fun, making the experience more meaningful. Rewards can be:

- Extra time with a parent or favorite person doing a preferred activity (e.g., a board game, outdoor play, time on the computer)
- Silly behavior from a parent (e.g., jumping in the pool fully clothed)
- A treat (e.g., a lollipop, favorite meal, or special dessert)
- Praise and affection
- A special outing (e.g., a trip to the movies)

Rewards are not bribes. A bribe is what we might try to give someone when we want her to do something that is of benefit to us. However, a reward is what we give to a person who has put effort into achieving something for herself. When using rewards for anxious individuals it is important that rewards are proportional. In other words, rewards need to match the level of difficulty or anxiety associated with the goal or challenge that is set. Going back to the example earlier of the goals/steps in overcoming a fear of dogs, we might allocate smaller level rewards such as choosing what's for dinner or deciding what everyone will watch on TV for smaller steps (e.g., Steps 1–3). Then we might allocate larger rewards such as a special treat or toy for more challenging steps (e.g., Steps 4–7). Finally, we would appoint the largest rewards such as going to the movies to the hardest steps (e.g., Steps 8–9). Therefore, the overall plan for goals toward overcoming a fear of dogs and the related rewards might look like Table 5.

Table 5	Sample Steps for Conquering a Fear of Dogs
Conquering a fear of dogs	
Goal/Step	**Reward**
1. Listen to someone read a book about dogs aloud.	Decide what everyone will watch on TV.
2. Look at still pictures of dogs on the Internet.	Choose what's for dinner.
3. Watch video footage of dogs on the Internet.	Stay up ten minutes past bedtime.
4. Stand outside the pet shop and look at dogs through the window.	Get an ice cream cone.
5. Visit a friend or relative who has a dog and watch the dog play outside (while standing inside).	Choose a DVD from the rental shop.
6. Stand outside and watch a dog while it is on a leash.	Go over to a friend's house.
7. Pat a dog on a leash.	Get a new book or computer game.
8. Play "catch" with a friend or relative's dog briefly for two minutes (with supervision or support from an adult).	Go out for a pizza.
9. Play with a friend or relative's dog for ten minutes.	Go out to a movie.

Again, it is helpful to remember that rewards need to be delivered immediately, i.e., as soon as the person carries out the set task. Therefore, you need to carefully plan when you will carry out the tasks of each step so that, as much as possible, the person engages in the activity right before you are ready to give the reward. It is also important to remember that rewards need to be given every time the person carries out the set task. Therefore, if a child practices Step 1 from Table 5 three times in a week, then she would also be allowed to choose what everyone watched on TV three times that week.

Once she has overcome her anxiety or conquered a step, then you can consider slowly fading out rewards so that the child does not come to expect a reward every time. From the example above, once a child is comfortable looking at dogs through the pet shop window, then you might fade out getting an ice cream cone every time by having ice cream available every second time, then every fourth, then every eighth, then not at all. Alternatively, you can explain to the child that rewards will now become like "random acts of kindness" in that she'll just never know when she'll get one. It could be tomorrow, it could be the next week, it could be two times in the same week! We will explore the idea of goal-setting again in much more detail in Chapter 8 when we look at how to develop "stepladders" in cognitive behavior therapy (CBT).

5. Emotion Coaching

While I would not encourage parents to spend too much time paying attention to their child's worries (see strategy #6 below, Planned Ignoring of Non-brave Behavior), it is important that parents clearly acknowledge when their child is feeling anxious or fearful. We have all experienced the difference it makes to us when someone notices that we feel uncomfortable and articulates this in a way that tells us that she really understands *exactly* how we feel. Usually, when we feel that someone understands us, we are more likely to follow any advice she gives us than if we feel that she cannot see our perspective. For example, if I was feeling petrified about seeing a spider in my house, I would be more likely to listen to advice about staying calm and getting rid of the spider if I first felt that my fear was acknowledged and understood rather than ignored or disregarded.

Emotion coaching is a term used to describe the process of clearly articulating to another person that you understand how she feels (Faber & Mazlish, 1980; Gottman, 1997). Essentially, it is a way of showing that you empathize or can truly "put yourself in someone's shoes." Emotion coaching involves describing for the person the emotions that you can see she is experiencing and why you think she might be feeling that way (Faber & Mazlish, 1980, Gottman, 1997). It is more than simply labeling an emotion briefly or telling a person that you "know how she feels" without substantiating this with any "evidence" that tells her that you do in fact understand her. For people with autism, emotion coaching is likely to be most effective for those who are higher functioning or have Asperger's disorder—who have broadly fluent language skills and better developed cognitive skills. According to Gottman (1997), the five key steps involved in emotion coaching are:

1. Being aware of the person's emotions
2. Recognizing emotional expression as an opportunity for intimacy and teaching
3. Listening empathetically and validating the person's feelings
4. Labeling emotions in words the person can relate to and understand
5. Helping the person to discover appropriate ways to solve a problem or deal with an upsetting situation

Examples of emotion coaching in relation to feelings of anxiety might include:

- *"You seem to be feeling quite worried about starting your homework. I guess you might be thinking that it seems too hard. Perhaps you are feeling a little overwhelmed by it, like there's too much hard work to get through and you're not really in the right mood to do it. Maybe we can work at it together."*

- *"I can see that you are feeling scared of visiting your cousin today because of her dog. You're probably thinking about the dog's teeth and her loud bark. It seems like you are worrying about whether the dog might bite you. I was wondering whether it might help if we try to stay close together when the dog is around."*

- *"It looks to me as though you're feeling a little lonely and maybe a bit scared about making friends at school. I'm wondering if you're thinking about how hard it can be to understand the other kids there and fit in with them. Maybe you're worried that the other kids at school will laugh at you or think you're weird. What if we plan out together how you might try to start a really short conversation tomorrow with one person whom you like at school?"*

- *"I can see that you've stopped studying for your exam so I'm guessing that you might be feeling a little overwhelmed by it all. I guess you might be worrying about how you'll possibly find the time to review the whole textbook before your exam this week when you still have other homework and school ac-*

tivities to complete. It looks as though you're ready to give up.
Maybe I could help you work on a timetable so that we can
organize how you can make time to get through the work."

- *"You're looking quite upset so I guess you must be feeling wor-*
  ried about tasting a new vegetable with your dinner. It looks
  as though you are scared about how it will feel in your mouth
  and that it might taste disgusting. What if we cut it up into
  smaller pieces and take some breaks in between bites?"

From the examples above you can see that you need to really
try to "put yourself in the other person's shoes" in order to be able to
speak sincerely to her about how she might be feeling. However, you
can also see that by articulating to her what she is feeling and why, you
end up in a better position to suggest tackling a problem rather than
just giving up or avoiding it altogether.

6. *Planned Ignoring of Non-brave Behavior*

As stated earlier, parents need to give more attention to brave behavior and less attention to non-brave behavior. This involves a technique
called "planned ignoring." Essentially, a parent briefly acknowledges that
the child may feel worried or anxious with words such as "I can see you
are feeling nervous about…" but then tries to move away from her child
once she has given a suggestion regarding what the child can do to cope
better. Emotion coaching (described above in strategy #5) can be used
to briefly acknowledge your child's feelings before using planned ignoring. Depending on the person's level of support needs and age, it might
be sensible to forewarn her that you will only acknowledge her anxiety
once before you expect her to try using her skills to cope. (Strategies to
help your child better recognize her own feelings of anxiety and to put
into place skills to cope are covered in detail in Chapter 8.) Ignoring or
reducing responses to behaviors such as repetitive questioning, checking,
fretting, and avoidance is critical in reducing anxiety. We need to show
the anxious person that we will give plenty of attention and reinforcement when she is brave, not when she is anxious.

Typically, when I discuss this strategy with parents, they tend to
think that they might seem too "harsh" or "tough" if they try to limit
non-brave behavior by walking away or limiting their response and at-

tention. They often state that they feel "guilty" not responding to their child when the child is fearful or distressed. Certainly, planned ignoring is one of the hardest techniques for a parent to adopt. It is natural for a parent to want to respond to every concern her child might have. However, planned ignoring is one of the most effective ways to clearly show a child that she is much better spending her energy being brave because less time and attention is given to her when she isn't coping. Gently remind yourself that you're not doing your child any favors by letting her fret. Remember, the objects or situations that most of us fear are usually innocuous or safe. This is no different for individuals with an ASD. Therefore:

- Avoid answering the child every time she repeatedly asks whether math is first, before reading groups at school that day.
- Avoid responding when a person with autism asks you to make sure all the dolls in her doll house face the same way.
- Limit affection and comfort when a child is having a tantrum because she lost at a board game.
- Avoid or limit conversation with a child or adolescent when she wants to discuss all the reasons why she doesn't want to do her math homework or start her assignment.
- Limit time spent trying to reason with a teenager with autism who seems anxious about giving a presentation in class and wants you to write a note to the teacher seeking a special exemption.

7. Model Brave Behavior

We can develop bravery and confidence in children by modeling that kind of behavior for them. The more we display bravery and confidence in our own actions, the more children are likely to pick up on this style of behavior as the better way to approach their own fears or worries. It is important that we model brave or confident behavior in a way that is obvious to the person with autism. That is, we might need to talk through our brave behavior as we display it or over-demonstrate it so that it is very clear. For example, we might say:

- *"I'm feeling a little worried about my meeting today because I have to speak in front of my team. But I'm going to stay calm and take some slow, deep breaths to help myself feel more relaxed and confident. I'm sure it will all be fine."*

- *"I'm a bit worried that Dad hasn't called yet to say he is coming home. I'll just tell myself that everything will be alright. Dad's been home late many times before and he's a good driver."*

- *"I can't seem to get my worried thoughts out of my head about all of the work I have to finish. Maybe I should take a break and go for a quick walk to try to clear away my worried thoughts. Yes, I think I'll do that now so that I can calm down on my own."*

- *"I really don't like the taste of sliced cheese. It feels disgusting in my mouth. But I'm going to be brave and break it up into smaller pieces and try a little bit at a time so that I get used to it."*

Video modeling might also be a helpful adjunct to the above suggestions. Parents can model examples of brave behavior on video and then play these back to help "coach" their child regarding how to approach a situation that concerns her. Similarly, it might be both a helpful and a fun exercise for younger children with autism to try to spot examples of brave behavior in cartoon characters, actors/actresses, or other celebrities that they relate to or like. Often, when we see people we admire engaging in brave behavior, we are likely to try to imitate them.

8. Role Reversal

We all know that children and adolescents like to have a turn at telling an adult what to do! By coaching Mom or Dad in what to do when he or she feels worried, the child with autism is more likely to take the same advice herself in order to continue to set a good example for her parent. Role reversal allows her to do this with a special focus on teaching an adult how to be more brave or confident. Perhaps think of it as a type of "reverse psychology." When we give a person extra control or responsibility over us to show or teach us what to do, she tends to take the task seriously. Consider some of the following ideas that you might use with children or adolescents:

For a child…"I'm not sure how to stop myself from thinking about my meeting tomorrow and talking in front of all those people. You're usually really good at being brave. Can you teach me what to do so that I can feel brave too?"

For a child..."I saw that scary dog today. I felt so worried that it would bite me and I started to panic. I've seen you taking some big breaths when you feel scared. Can you show me what you do? I think that might help me feel more confident next time I have to walk near that dog."

For an adolescent..."I noticed that you were really confident when you started your homework this afternoon. I've got lots of work to get through tonight. I'm feeling overwhelmed about it. What did you do today to help get motivated to begin? Can you show me so that I can see if it works for me too?"

For an adolescent... "I've been thinking a lot about getting everything ready for the party next week and I just don't seem to feel confident that it will all get done. You seem pretty good at staying calm when you have lots of school work and assignments to get through. What do you tell yourself to help you get it done? Maybe it will work for me too."

The key with role reversal is asking for help, such that parents put themselves in the apprentice role. In turn, the parent boosts the child or adolescent's confidence and sense of competence in giving the parent help with being brave. Just as was discussed for rewarding brave behavior, it is important that you put effort into finding or creating opportunities for the child or adolescent to coach you. You might not truly believe that your son or daughter is the best person to tell you or teach you how to be confident; however, you might be pleasantly surprised how your child can rise to the occasion when she feels that she is in charge of an adult, especially her parent. Find quiet, special "parent-child" time to sit down and ask your son or daughter for his or her feedback and ideas. Scheduling the time like you would schedule a special meeting or appointment is a good way to help your child take the activity more seriously and feel as though you truly value her input.

9. Allocate Responsibilities and Encourage Independence

As discussed above, it is important to focus attention on bravery, not fear. By encouraging people with autism to give something their best shot or take on a task alone, we can help them learn that they can do it. We show them that they do not always need to rely on adult support to feel comfortable or safe. The best way to foster independence is to find or create opportunities within the home where the child can take on an extra job or responsibility that she can complete alone. It does not matter how simple the task is, so long as the parent reinforces and praises the fact that the person has shown bravery or confidence in completing the task alone—without assistance. If you think it helpful, you can walk your child through the task or activity first so that she feels comfortable with what is expected of her. Some key areas that might be targeted for people to develop more independence include:

- Asking a young child to be in charge of putting a small selection of toys away on her own.
- Asking a child to be in charge of planning the Saturday evening activities every other week on her own.
- Asking a child to be in charge of choosing what's for dinner each Wednesday night and picking out the recipe on her own.
- Asking an adolescent to be in charge of planning the evening TV shows on her own so that it is fair for each family member.
- Asking an adolescent to take control of organizing the weekly grocery list before the next big grocery shop.

From the examples above, you can see that the tasks are usually just daily, routine activities that the child or adolescent is probably quite capable of doing without any feelings of anxiety. However, the point is to try to find easy tasks that she feels comfortable trying or doing unassisted so that it is easier for you to find opportunities to reward or encourage her confidence and/or independence in doing them. That is, we want to set the child up to succeed. It is important that we place more emphasis on success and confidence in the person than perfection in completing the task. Therefore, we should avoid correcting the child if she puts the toys away without assistance but does so in a way that is not how you might do it. At times, parents might need to "bite their lips" and sacrifice a perfectly ordered house for the sake of building confidence in their son or daughter. If you try to choose tasks where you do not currently see confidence and independence, then you will have a much harder job finding opportunities to reward bravery. Remember, if we start with frequently rewarding an individual with autism for her bravery in the simplest of tasks, then she is more likely to apply herself independently to tasks that are genuinely challenging or fear-provoking. Also, when a person sees that she is able to take on more tasks independently, she is more likely to feel better about herself, i.e., to have higher self-esteem.

10. Allow and Encourage Mistakes

Understandably, sometimes parents of children with special needs can be particularly cautious about allowing their children to make mistakes or fail at a task. They might think that life for a person with autism is already challenging enough without experiencing further mistakes or challenges that the parent could help avoid or prevent. For example, parents I have worked with choose to avoid play dates and social gatherings (e.g., birthday parties) in case their children with autism struggle to fit in with the other children present and end up feeling like they "failed."

It is, of course, critical that we support people with autism in a way that sets them up for success—not failure. However, if we go out of our way to prevent them from experiencing mistakes or challenges, then we might also be preventing them from learning how to cope and ultimately how to improve their skills. For example, if a parent allows her child to engage in a play date or social gathering knowing that the child might "get it wrong" socially, then there is a greater chance that the parent and child will also learn how to cope and what to do next time. More specifically, if a parent allows her child to go to a birthday party and the child struggles to engage well socially by dominating the play or refusing to join in, then despite the challenge, the parent and child have good data about what to do differently next time. This might include looking someone in the eye when greeting her, taking turns for longer, offering a toy to another child, or asking another child to join in play. Parents can use a range of approaches such as video modeling, role playing, on the spot coaching, and social stories to help teach and practice these social skills. By persisting and practicing the required social skills, the parent and child learn to stay in a challenging social situation and cope, rather than avoid it. Essentially, practicing any skills will always involve making errors; otherwise we will never be able to reach a stage where we can display them successfully.

Allowing mistakes does not mean setting the person up to fail. It means limiting the attempts one might make to avoid mistakes or challenges. Some examples might include:

- Allowing a child to join the soccer team at her request even though you know that she might end up kicking the ball in the wrong direction or displaying poor motor coordination skills.
- Encouraging a child to attend a birthday party where team games and competitions might be involved, knowing that coping with winning and losing is an area of weakness for the child.
- Permitting an adolescent to join the school debate team at her request even though you believe that she might make errors in presenting a clear and sequential argument.
- Suggesting that an adolescent has a go at phoning a school peer to ask them to go and see a movie even though you know there is a chance that the peer might say no.
- Taking the eraser away to prevent a child from repeatedly rubbing out her errors on her math worksheet and replacing them with the correct responses. This way, she does not send "perfect" results back to the teacher, falsely indicating that she is fully competent.

I am sure that parents might read the above examples and feel that it would be too tough to allow their child to enter a situation where she is likely to make mistakes. However, it is more important for parents to encourage and reward their child for her efforts in "having a go" and learning to cope than it is to prevent the child from experiencing a mistake. After all, life for all of us is full of mistakes. Even if your child does not seem to want to accept the idea of "going for it" and potentially making a mistake, it is still important that you encourage her to do so.

There are no fixed rules regarding how much to push your child. As the expert on your child, only you can determine that. However, it might be possible to insist on her trying something and preventing her from backing out if you have set the task up to be manageable—that is, if you have started with an activity that is relatively mild in terms of how anxious the child might feel if she makes a mistake (strategy # 3 on goal setting could help you). Similarly, using strategies like emotion coaching (see strategy #5 above) might also assist in showing the child that you understand how she feels, thereby helping her to feel more supported in her anxiety so she is less likely to back out.

11. Schedule "Worry Time"

It seems ironic but it is helpful to allocate a special time for "worry" in order to reduce it! Sometimes people who experience anxiety talk repeatedly about their worries, raising concerns about future dangers or "what will happen if...?" Often, parents will report that they are exhausted by their child discussing worries and fears over and over again or repeatedly asking the parent for reassurance. It is when worries seem like they are taking over conversation and, therefore, much of parents' time that we need to set some clear limits on it. "Worry time" is all about setting limits on worries. Scheduling a specific, regular (e.g., daily) time slot wherein worries can be thought about, discussed, and problem-solved within a limited time period can be helpful in reducing anxiety for three reasons:

1. Setting a regular time to discuss worries or fears can help reassure the child that her problems can be discussed and addressed. That is, it can be relieving for her to know there is a special time slot allocated to trying to resolve her fears or anxieties.

2. Setting a clear time also helps to set limits on the anxious person. Specifically, by setting a regular worry time slot, we are, in turn, preventing her from using up all other time slots, i.e., any other time in the day to discuss her worries. You'd be surprised how quickly someone might lose the urge to discuss her worries whenever they arise if she knows she can rely on a regular time slot to do so.

3. Because worry time is scheduled, it tends to occur when the person is calmer and thinking more rationally as opposed to trying to solve a fear or worry in the very instance when the person is feeling most anxious. That is, there is more chance that the worry can actually be resolved because the person is more likely to be approaching worry time with a clear or open mind.

Here are some steps to help you implement worry time at home with your anxious son or daughter with autism. As applies to emotion coaching, worry time is most suitable to people with high functioning autism or Asperger's disorder.

Step 1: Make a regular time slot called something like "worry time," "thinking time," or "problem solving" time with the anxious person. It is very important that the time slot is set at the same time each day rather than a time that varies from day to day or week to week. Usually, ten to fifteen minutes per day is a good amount of time. It is also important that you pick a time when you are both likely to be free from other distractions.

Step 2: Create a list or "agenda" for worry time. You might put this on the kitchen fridge or bulletin board so that the anxious person can simply jot down any worries on it that she wants to discuss during worry time. If and when your child brings up a concern to you and wants to discuss it, don't become drawn into a worry session right then and there. Instead direct her to her worry list to jot it down (or explain that you will do this for her if she is unable). A list is very important in allowing the person to let go of worries or fears as they occur throughout the day. For example, if I began to worry about meeting a deadline at work, then, rather than cutting into my current activity and getting caught up in my fears and worries, I could write "work deadlines" on my worry list. This way I can get on with my current task knowing that the worry will be addressed later during worry time.

Step 3: When worry time arrives, sit down with the anxious child and determine which items from the worry list will be discussed. You might be able to cover them all in ten to fifteen minutes. However, if not, then you will need to ask the person to choose from the list. Whatever is not addressed in that worry time is then carried forward to the next worry time slot the next day. Worry time is not extended beyond the allocated time limit.

Step 4: During worry time, allow the person the opportunity to discuss the full extent of her worry. If relevant or possible, try to help her work out some practical steps to try to address or resolve her worry or fear.

Step 5: If the child is a concrete or visual learner, use a timer or clock to mark the ten or fifteen minutes of worry time and to show clearly when worry time is over.

Step 6: Once the time is up, wrap up worry time. You can do so by praising your child for her participation and re-confirming the next worry time slot. It is imperative that both the parent and the anxious child do not discuss anything further about the worry until the following worry time the next day. Similarly, it is also important that you don't model any fretting yourself outside of worry time. Therefore, as much as possible, refrain from too much "checking in," questioning, or seeking reassurance from your child as to her anxiety levels at other times.

Anxiety Prevention

All of the strategies outlined above can be implemented by parents not only to manage existing anxiety in their child with autism but also to *prevent* it from occurring or getting worse. In other words, you shouldn't wait until a person is highly anxious to try to implement the "indirect treatments" outlined above.

One tool that has been developed at my center for preventing anxiety for all parents and children, not specifically for children with autism, is a story book called, "Wally the Worried Wallaby" (Chalfant & Kyngdon, 2008). The story is about a wallaby (a type of kangaroo for those readers less familiar with Australian fauna) who is very fearful of dogs because of concerns about the germs they might carry. The story describes how, with the help of a confident koala named "Carli," Wally learns to overcome

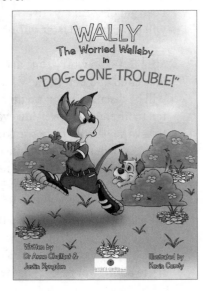

his fear of dogs via small steps. The book can be read to or with a child. There is a separate parent guide with ten exercises to help parents work on many of the strategies described above with their child. The aim of the book is for parents to help raise awareness in their child about worries and emotions such as fear. Another aim is for parents to work on the prescribed activities just as frequently as they would other fun activities with their child (e.g., crafts, coloring, card games). In doing so, the book and parent guide help parents to teach their child to develop confidence and resilience. The more confident and resilient a child is, the less likely she is to experience an anxiety or mood problem later on in her life.

In Summary

- When someone is fearful or anxious, we are presented with a dilemma regarding how best to support her: Do we encourage her to be brave and face her fear or do we permit avoidance of the feared object or situation?
- Encouraging bravery involves short-term challenges. Usually when we encourage someone to face her fears we might see an increase in resistant and challenging behavior.
- Alternatively, permitting avoidance of a feared object or situation involves short term relief because there is no emphasis on facing an uncomfortable situation.
- In the longer term, it is healthier for parents to encourage bravery in their child with an ASD by helping her to face her fears.
- The more we support someone avoiding a fear, the more anxious she will become.
- Avoidance increases anxiety because it limits the number of opportunities we have to face the feared object or situation and, therefore, learn that we can probably cope if we remain in the situation for long enough.
- There are both direct and indirect treatments we can use to manage and reduce anxiety. Parents can use indirect "treatments" by:
  - ❑ Praising bravery
  - ❑ Giving extra attention to brave and/or independent behavior

- ❏ Setting goals
- ❏ Proportional rewards
- ❏ Emotion coaching
- ❏ Ignoring non-brave behavior
- ❏ Modeling brave behavior
- ❏ Role reversal
- ❏ Allocating responsibilities
- ❏ Allowing mistakes
- ❏ Scheduling "worry time"

- It is important to focus on preventing anxiety from occurring in the first place rather than only trying to manage it once it arises. Some simple resources are now being developed to help parents teach their children about worries from an early age and to help them develop skills that build resilience.

- Resources, like the book "Wally the Worried Wallaby," help young children develop awareness about how to remain confident. Better anxiety awareness and skills to combat anxiety early in life may prevent anxiety or other mood difficulties occurring later in life. (See Appendices B and C.)

Treating Anxiety:
Indirect Treatments for Use by Preschools, Schools, and Clinics

Kyle and the Maskell Family

Kyle's parents asked me to attend a school meeting with them regarding Kyle's school support. They were concerned that Kyle was spending each recess and lunch period in a "passive play room" that the school had set up for students who were not comfortable being out on the playground. They felt that while the passive play room had been helpful as a starting point for Kyle in reducing his social anxiety, it was now time to move beyond this strategy. They believed that both Kyle and the school teachers might be relying on it too heavily rather than encouraging Kyle to spend time on the playground with students his age. Most of the children in the passive play room were younger than Kyle or had their own special needs. His parents wanted to ensure that Kyle was given opportunities to develop his social skills with the students in his year and his class, almost all of whom spent their recess and lunch periods participating in outdoor play.

Kyle's parents believed that Kyle had the social skills to participate with his same age peers, despite his reported social anxiety. He had been to numerous social skills classes and could "talk the talk." He could correctly answer all of the questions and participate effectively in all of the structured activities within the social skills groups based on turn taking, initiating play, joining in, and keeping play going. What Kyle was lacking was "hands on" or "live" practice of these learned skills within the school playground context.

When Kyle's parents and I met with Kyle's school principal, classroom teacher, special education teacher, and teacher's aide it seemed clear that the school was reluctant to move Kyle out of the passive play room, even for one recess or lunch period per week. They also seemed quite *hesitant to want to introduce a playground-based social skills program to support Kyle's transition to the playground with his same age peers. Rather, they stated that, if Kyle was comfortable in the passive playroom, then they did not want to disrupt him or create anxiety for him by suggesting he try to play in a new environment. Moreover, the school staff reported that they felt somewhat anxious and overwhelmed themselves. They described that they might not have the appropriate skills or resources to create a playground program for Kyle.*

Discussion occurred regarding how to break this process down into smaller, more manageable steps for both Kyle and the school. Suggestions included that Kyle work individually with either the special education teacher or the teacher's aide on some key phrases to use when trying to enter a game on the playground; that a practice schedule be arranged for Kyle to begin to implement these skills once per week as a first step; that a check-off and reward system be set up for a teacher to sign at the end of the play period to note that Kyle had completed the set activity; and that a reward system be implemented to immediately reward Kyle for his brave efforts in being on the playground with his classmates.

Despite my suggestions, as well as the family's belief that Kyle was capable of practicing his social skills with students his age and the fact that his time in the passive playroom was predominantly spent teaching other younger students how to play chess (i.e., he was not "socializing" in a reciprocal way), the school refused to implement the recommended playground program. They stated that their main concern was that Kyle would become anxious or worried about being on the playground, even if he knew the social skills to use. They were not prepared to push him beyond his "comfort zone." This concern on the part of the school staff permeated their approach to other school events. The school arranged special exemptions for Kyle from attending the school field days as well as the end-of-year school concerts.

Understandably, the thought of extra time or resources in setting up a playground support program or other support programs for the bigger school events might have seemed daunting for the school staff. Their concern for Kyle's anxiety was admirable. However, ultimately Kyle continued to be isolated from his same age peers as, outside of class time, he had no interaction with them. Furthermore, the more Kyle spent time in the passive play room engaging with younger children or other students with special needs, the less inclined his same-age peers were to want to socialize with him as they began to associate him with the younger students and as a child with some kind of "problem." The less inclined Kyle's peers were to interact with him, the more isolated he felt and the more anxious he became about socializing with them.

Ultimately, the family chose to move Kyle out of the school and into a new mainstream environment. A transition program was set up including a peer education program for the class ahead of Kyle's attendance at the school so that his classmates were aware of his special needs and how best to include him in their play. Some key students were asked to become "buddies" for Kyle during recess and lunch periods. The playground program suggested to the first school was also implemented. Kyle was also given special roles to oversee at major school events. For example, he was appointed time-keeper for the school sporting events.

Now Kyle has begun to establish some reciprocal friendships with other students in his class. He reports feeling happier, and he has begun to spend more time with his classmates outside of school via play dates and sleepovers.

The Common Anxiety Dilemma for Teachers and Healthcare Professionals

In the example of Kyle above, it is clear that the classroom teacher and the other school administrators faced a dilemma regarding how best to manage Kyle's anxiety:

Option 1:

Do they try to alleviate Kyle's anxiety by allowing him to keep going to the passive play room? The passive play room for more comfortable lunch periods seemed like a manageable long-term option for the school. It's understandable that having a room within the school where Kyle could occupy himself with limited adult supervision would have seemed more logistically appealing for the school. The school needed to use less staff and related resources trying to manage successful lunch time games and interactions with the other children. Also, Kyle might have felt less anxious there because he did not have to participate in playground games with his peers.

Similarly, should the school allow Kyle to opt out of attending major school events such as the field days and end of year school assemblies and concerts because these might be too anxiety provoking for him? This option would also seem much easier for the school to manage. There would be no need to have special support plans or people in place for Kyle. Therefore, there would be fewer requirements to allocate extra time, money, and related resources to organizing such support.

Kyle's family's situation is very common among families of people with autism. In the author's years of experience consulting with schools, it seems that one of the hardest suggestions for a school to follow up and implement is that of a lunch time play group or club to support the needs of a child with autism. In particular, schools tend to be easily overwhelmed and perhaps somewhat anxious about how they would allocate time and resources to the social support of a student with an ASD. In an age when there is less and less funding available to schools for individuals with disabilities, it is understandable that schools are worried about how best to make use of the limited resources and staff they may have.

Option 2:

Do the classroom teacher and other school professionals try to engage Kyle in the activities he fears or the situations where he feels uncomfortable, as was the choice of the second school? This option involved many more demands on the classroom teacher and other school staff at first. Extra time, effort, and people were required to arrange appropriate support for Kyle during major school events, not to mention extra time and work spent in preparing resources (e.g., visual schedules) for Kyle ahead of the events so that he understood exactly what to expect and what might be expected of him. Then there was the possibility of managing challenging behavior from Kyle if he began to worry or panic when attending large school events or during a lunch time when he might misunderstand another child or take over during a game. In summary, this option probably involved dealing with not only more challenging behavior from Kyle, but also involved coping with more logistical demands on the school.

In the long term, although initially more difficult, it is more effective for Kyle to learn to experience and subsequently cope with situations that make him feel anxious rather than avoid them. Just as we explored in Chapter 5 on parenting anxious children, it is important that students and/or clients are encouraged to face their fears rather than be allowed to engage in "safety seeking" behavior or avoidance. As we did in Chapter 5, in the current chapter we will explore this dilemma for teachers and other professionals who work with children with autism. Likewise, a number of strategies that teachers and other professionals can use to help manage anxious behavior in their school, clinic, or other support settings will be outlined. These strategies address the way we can implement support techniques, develop resources, or adjust the child's environment to help increase the child's resilience and boost his self-confidence, thereby indirectly reducing his anxiety. Some of the strategies discussed are similar to those outlined for parents in Chapter 5. However, given that home, school, and clinic settings are very different from one another, it is important to consider the application of these strategies separately for each setting.

What Makes Professionals Anxious about Working with People "On the Spectrum?"

Autism is certainly a frequently discussed topic within health and education; however, compared with other childhood difficulties, there still seems to be little understanding of autism. Moreover, while scientific research has improved significantly, there are still many misconceptions about autism as well as many unsupported treatments that are marketed to people with autism, their families, and those who work with them. Consequently, in the author's experience of consulting to various schools and health organizations, it seems that many professionals see working with autism as a specialty and, therefore, feel anxious and overwhelmed about working with an individual on the spectrum. For example, many teachers, school principals, speech pathologists, psychologists, pediatricians, and psychiatrists report feeling unsuitably trained or ill-equipped to work with people with autism, preferring to arrange for them to be placed in another classroom or school setting, or attempting to refer them onto another healthcare professional.

Professionals' Worries and Misconceptions about Working with Someone with an ASD

Myth: *All people with an ASD have very challenging behavior.*

Many professionals have come to associate autism with oppositional and challenging behavior. This is a false premise or wrong assumption. Indeed, the author sees many children with autism who have been overdiagnosed with other co-morbid labels such as conduct disorder (CD) and oppositional defiant disorder (ODD). Consequently, many professionals fear that working with a person with autism will necessitate having to cope with more tantrums, lashing out, and possible aggressive behavior. In reality, not all people with autism have challenging behavior, just as not all people with autism have a special interest in the same object or subject. You may have heard the saying, "When you have met one individual child with autism, then you have met one individual with autism." Essentially, this means that each person with an ASD can present quite differently despite their similar language, social skills, and creative play difficulties.

Myth: *You need to be a specialist to work with someone with an ASD.*

Professionals such as teachers and psychologists frequently tell me that they are anxious about working with a person with autism because they do not have the specialized skills or training to do so. Moreover, they often suggest that mainstream behavior or learning support strategies are not appropriate because a person with autism has a unique thinking and learning style and, therefore, must automatically require a different approach. That is, in general, there seems to be a misconception that when working with a client with autism, you cannot apply strategies that you know work with other groups of people or with typically developing individuals. Rather, there seems to be a belief that we need to invent something new or different. Unfortunately—and partly as a result of this kind of misconception—there are a plethora of "alternative" approaches with interesting acronyms that purport all sorts of treatments and "cures" for people with autism without a shred of sound scientific research to support their efficacy. Yet, because there is a belief that an individual with an ASD requires a unique treatment approach, vulnerable families are sold these treatments as the only way to really support their son or daughter.

In reality, often the most evidence-based and scientifically supported strategies for working with people with autism are not new or "specialized." Rather, they tend to be the same strategies that we have been applying for decades to other groups of children and adults with language, social, learning, or emotional difficulties. For example, in the field of psychology and psychiatry, cognitive behavior therapy (CBT) (discussed at length in Chapter 8) was first developed in the 1970's by Aaron Beck (e.g., Beck, 1976). CBT has been applied for the past three decades to treat a wide range of mental health and emotional difficulties in both children and adults including Anxiety Disorders, Depression, Bipolar Disorder, Eating Disorders, Post Traumatic Stress Disorder, and Psychotic Disorders including Schizophrenia. Most recently we have begun to see clinicians applying CBT programs or strategies to their work with children with autism. For example, TEACCH (Treatment and Education of Autistic and related Communication-handicapped CHildren), based at the University of North Carolina, provides evidence-based services for individuals of all ages and skill levels with autism spectrum disorders. Its learning support strategies are based on a cognitive-behavioral approach (Mesibov, Shea, & Schopler, 2005). Similarly, clinicians and researchers are beginning to demonstrate that CBT can be applied to people with autism as a means of addressing their social, communication, and anxiety difficulties (e.g., Chalfant, Rapee & Carroll, 2006; Sofronoff, Attwood & Hinton, 2005; White et al., 2010). Therefore, rather than trying to invent new treatment programs or therapies (at times with little scientific research to support their use), it has been demonstrated that we can simply apply existing ones to new groups of people or adapt current programs for use with new populations.

Myth: *Working with someone with an ASD requires too much extra work.*

Understandably, teachers may worry about the extra work that they believe will be involved in teaching a person with autism, when they already have a classroom of twenty to thirty children to work with and manage. They might imagine extra hours spent preparing visual cues, managing behavior, and adjusting curriculum. However, effective teaching techniques for children with autism are usually the same as those that work well for typically developing children. Specifically, they are usually common-sense, structured teaching techniques such as breaking work down into smaller steps, using visuals to support oral instructions, and using positive reinforcement and rewards for effort to help motivate students to remain on task. Therefore, the extra work envisaged might not be as labor intensive as some teachers believe.

Myth: *The other students will suffer.*

Professionals have raised concerns with the author during consultations about "spoiling it" for the other children in the classroom or clinical setting by including a person with autism. For example, teachers have raised concerns about taking a student with autism along on a school fieldtrip. They fear that the child's behavior or need for more individual supervision might take time and focus away from the other children in the class or detract from the other children's enjoyment. Again, while these concerns seem reasonable, it is highly unlikely that supporting a child with autism well would take up so much time and energy that there would be none left over for the other students. As described above, all children benefit from structured teaching, clear preparation for activities such as fieldtrips, and organized classrooms. Therefore, a teacher who applies structured teaching methods across the board (regardless of the type of children he has in his class) is usually much more likely to have a class full of students who have had successful and enjoyable experiences during activities such as fieldtrips rather than a group of disgruntled students who feel overlooked.

Encourage Bravery or Permit Avoidance?

Just as there was a dilemma for parents discussed in Chapter 5, in the example of Kyle above, the school professionals were facing a dilemma: Do they exclude Kyle from activities that they believe might be too anxiety-provoking for him and perhaps too anxiety-provoking for them in terms of managing him? Alternatively, do they encourage Kyle to participate and arrange support for him accordingly? Essentially the dilemma faced by Kyle's classroom teacher and the other school professionals reflects a broader issue often faced by education and healthcare professionals who work with people with autism and their families: Do we encourage the person to face his fears or avoid what he is fearful of? Table 6 shows some common examples of dilemmas that professionals face regarding whether to encourage bravery or permit avoidance. It is likely that you have been asked these questions yourselves by parents you work with or that you have faced these issues within your own classroom or clinic.

From Table 6 you can see that although the topic area might be different, essentially the dilemma remains the same. So, just as was discussed for parents in Chapter 5, is it better for professionals to encourage bravery or to permit avoidance? Again, both options have their advantages and disadvantages. Therefore, just as was reviewed in Chapter 5, perhaps the best way to answer this dilemma is to look at the likely outcomes of encouraging bravery vs. those of permitting avoidance and then decide which are better.

Table 6	Common Anxiety Dilemmas for Professionals	
Issue/topic	**Encouraging bravery**	**Permitting avoidance**
Group work	Do I encourage the child to participate in group activities for gradually longer periods of time?	Do I allow the child to sit out of group activities such as reading groups or turn-taking games because he struggles to participate and it might make it unpleasant for the other children in the group?
Play time	Do I encourage the child to stay on the playground and help him find ways to join in established groups?	Do I allow the child to use the library each recess and lunch time because he is more comfortable in the quieter area reading a book or using the computer?
Winning and losing	Do I try to teach the student to cope with losing or not being first all the time?	Do I avoid games where the student might lose or situations where he is not first, e.g., forming lines when entering and leaving the classroom?
School assemblies	Do I insist that the child attends and participates in the assembly along with his class for gradually longer periods of time?	Do I exempt the child from school assemblies because of the over-stimulation and sensory difficulties it might cause him?
School fieldtrips	Do I suggest that the child attends the school fieldtrips?	Do I suggest that the child not attend fieldtrips because he might feel uncomfortable in a new environment and his behavior might be harder to manage in a public place?
Making mistakes/ perfectionism	Do I teach the child to make mistakes and cope?	Do I allow the child to re-start his work each time he makes a mistake so that he does not become disappointed with himself?

(continued on next page)

Changes in routine	Do I try to introduce more changes into the child's routines so that he learns to cope with change?	Do I try to ensure that there are no changes to the child's routines or that all changes are forewarned so that he is always comfortable and knows what to expect of each situation he experiences?

Encouraging Bravery

By encouraging bravery in a school or clinic context, it is likely that the child will become distressed or anxious initially. For example, if we encourage an anxious child who is fearful of presenting news in front of the class to stand up and deliver even a small piece of information to his classmates, then he is likely at first to experience distress or anxiety. However, as discussed in Chapter 5, we know from scientific research over many years that if an anxious person regularly experiences the object of his anxiety, then his initial fear response will eventually shift to one of coping. Therefore, the more we expose clients (at preschools, schools, or clinics) to objects or situations that might make them feel anxious, but are otherwise safe, the more likely they are to eventually learn that they can cope. The example below of Micaela is a case in point.

Micaela, five years of age

Micaela is an included kindergarten student who has a strong fear of making mistakes. She avoids attempting school work that she describes as "too hard." In particular, she avoids any work involving the alphabet including reading, writing letters, or completing classroom drills on the alphabet and the various sounds that each letter makes. When presented with work that she believes is too hard, she makes loud, repetitive noises, screams "No!", or talks over the teacher as if trying to block out the task instructions. She also says things like, "It's too hard," "I don't know," or "Go now" when she wants to put a quick end to a task. It is important to note that Micaela is actually extremely familiar with letters and possesses literacy skills well beyond most children her age.

With support from Micaela's behavior therapist, the classroom teacher chose the option of encouraging bravery rather than allowing Micaela exemption from literacy tasks. For example, the teacher decided to ignore any yelling or comments made by Micaela about the difficulty of literacy tasks or any attempts she made to speak over the classroom teacher. The teacher then broke up the literacy tasks into smaller segments of work for Micaela to complete. For example, if the class was completing a worksheet requiring copying sentences, then Micaela was presented with smaller amounts of the same work as well as other letter-based work such as coloring in or cutting out letter shapes. This was to more fully immerse Micaela in experiencing letter-based tasks. A reward system was also implemented for any attempts Micaela made toward completing the smaller literacy tasks.

As Micaela became more and more used to completing the shorter literacy tasks, the task length and complexity was increased along with the type of rewards given. Moreover, the reward or incentive system was also used to reward other "incidental" examples of "brave" behavior from Micaela including putting up her hand in class to offer information, answering a question in front of her peers, or completing a task that she enjoyed (e.g., art) independently. Eventually, after approximately two months, Micaela was able to complete the same literacy tasks as her peers without worry or distress regarding the task difficulty and whether or not she might make a mistake.

The example above highlights two points. First, the classroom teacher experienced short-term difficulties in trying to encourage Micaela to complete literacy work and face her fears. Encouraging bravery toward making errors is usually associated with an initial increase in challenging behavior. Second, with persistence, the classroom teacher was able to shift Micaela's initial fear response to one where she could tolerate both the task and the possibility of errors.

Permitting Avoidance

By permitting avoidance, people are less likely to become distressed or anxious in the short term. For example, if we allow children with autism to avoid being on the playground at recess or lunch time, then they are less likely to have an opportunity to feel socially anxious or uncomfortable among their school peers. However, as scientific research over many years has shown, if someone who is socially anxious regularly avoids interaction with other people, then, ultimately, each time he is in a social situation, his level of social anxiety will increase—not decrease. The increase in anxiety will be because he will have had fewer opportunities to see that he might cope in the presence of other people his age. Basically, the less he is exposed to social situations that might make him feel anxious, but are otherwise safe, the less he is able to learn that those situations might be manageable. Therefore, the more likely he is to feel even more anxious and insecure the next time he meets other people. Consider the example of another client:

Nathan, ten years old

Nathan said he felt worried about being on the playground at recess and lunch time because he felt unsure of how to initiate play with his peers. He worried that the other students did not want to play with him. He believed that they thought of him as "weird." I recall him telling me, "Making friends is harder than you think. I'm always scared they'll yell 'No!'" Consequently, Nathan would avoid the playground each day. He was given special permission to use the school library during lunch and recess. Indeed, an area was virtually reserved for him to use each day where he could read quietly or play a computer game.

Nathan's social worries seemed to increase over time. In class, when asked if he wanted to present news or answer a question in front of his classmates, he would refuse, feeling anxious and believing that, if he responded, his classmates would laugh at him. Unfortunately, the extra difficulty for Nathan was that the more he was exempt from participating in class activities, the more "weird" he did seem to all the other children. They did not understand why he did not want to talk in front of them and why he was given special permission not to do so. Therefore, the school's choice of permitting avoidance seemed to make life more challenging for Nathan rather than supporting him, as was their intention.

Nathan's case highlights two points. First, every time he was allowed to use the library rather than the playground, he felt comfort and relief from not having to interact with his peers; that is, his anxiety level dropped. However, in the longer term, Nathan's avoidance actually served to isolate him further from his peers—not only reinforcing his own faulty thinking that he was not good enough socially to join in with them but also allowing his peers to become confused and perhaps somewhat "put off" by his behavior. Second, just as in the example earlier of Kyle, the school's attempts to support Nathan by allowing him special access to the library and exempting him from some socially challenging classroom activities served to increase rather than decrease his social anxiety in the long term. Since Nathan had less and less opportunity to engage socially, he became more and more convinced that he could not cope if he had to interact with his peers.

Short Term Pain; Long Term Gain

In Chapter 5, we explored the longer term benefits for a person who can learn to be brave and face his fears. Specifically, benefits such as developing better coping skills, greater independence, and ultimately greater self-confidence and self-esteem were outlined. However, there are also benefits for those professionals who work with anxious children who, themselves, might feel anxious about their ability to support a person with autism.

A recent example I experienced of the benefits to professionals in helping children face fears was concerning Mr. Smith, a client's third grade teacher.

Mr. Smith, third grade teacher

My client Tyrone entered Mr. Smith's class in a mainstream school after three years in a support classroom within a special school for children with autism. Consequently, both Mr. Smith and Tyrone's parents were very nervous about how well Tyrone would transition into full-time inclusive education as well as how well Mr. Smith would be able to cope with the possible demands of a student with autism in his class. At first, Mr. Smith requested that a full-time aide be assigned to support Tyrone while he continued to work with the rest of the class. In this way, he later agreed, he seemed to be avoiding having to work closely with Tyrone. Moreover, at first, Tyrone was allowed to get away with behaviors that Tyrone knew were considered unacceptable at home, in public, or in my clinic. In particular, if Tyrone was presented with a task that he could complete but preferred not to because of the effort involved, then he would sit under his desk and ignore Mr. Smith. At first, Mr. Smith allowed Tyrone to engage in this behavior, believing that he might cause Tyrone more anxiety if he pushed him to get back to work.

During my first consultation with Mr. Smith, he indicated that he was very anxious about having Tyrone in his classroom. He said that he did not feel at all capable of teaching him and suggested that he did not have any skills to work with children with special needs. He had prepared a list of almost twenty different incidents and challenges within the first few weeks of school where he requested my input and direction regarding how he could have better managed. What struck me about Mr. Smith was that it seemed he had "given up on himself" before he had really begun. He was lacking self-confidence regarding his own skills despite the fact that he had been an excellent classroom teacher for almost twenty years and had a wealth of experience regarding managing challenging behavior. It seemed that the word "autism" had sent shivers up his spine, rendering him a nervous wreck about how well he could manage the class with Tyrone in it.

As we discussed each of the incidents that Mr. Smith had listed, it became clear that he had handled Tyrone extremely well or certainly had a clear sense of what strategies might work best next time. As a brief exercise, I asked Mr. Smith to temporarily forget Tyrone's diagnosis of autism and instead imagine that Tyrone was simply another member of the class. I then asked him to consider and talk about what strategies, learning support measures, or behavior management programs he would consider using for a child with Tyrone's intelligence and weaknesses. He instantly responded with suggestions such as visual supports, breaking harder tasks down into smaller segments for Tyrone to complete one step at a time, the use of incentive systems to be matched to segmented tasks, buddying Tyrone with students who displayed good, on-task behaviors, and allocating small but "special" responsibilities to Tyrone to increase his participation within the class and raise his social profile (e.g., putting him in charge of the book corner). I then suggested that perhaps these strategies might well be suitable for Tyrone too. He seemed surprised that he might actually be capable of teaching Tyrone in this way. When we next spoke a few months later, Mr. Smith was a much calmer and more confident man. He indicated that he had few concerns regarding Tyrone's support and had, in fact, suggested that the aide take on a more indirect role within the classroom (e.g., helping to prepare relevant visual resources) while he taught the entire class including Tyrone.

What my conversations with Mr. Smith highlighted again was the importance of facing fears and believing that one is capable of coping rather than avoiding challenges. Moreover, Mr. Smith's example emphasizes the idea that a change in his teaching strategies was not required. That is, he simply needed to apply tried and true strategies to a new student and dive in rather than convince himself that because Tyrone has autism he required a "new bag of tricks."

Avoidance Increases Anxiety in Your Student or Client

As was discussed in Chapter 4, it is critical that, as professionals, we do not indirectly increase a person's anxiety by helping him avoid what he fears, even though we are trying to support our student or client. By avoiding the objects or situations that an anxious person with autism might fear, we are essentially preventing him from learning that he might actually be able to cope.

Going back to Table 6 and the common dilemmas that education and healthcare professionals often discuss with me, it might now be clearer that it is better in the longer term to take the option of encouraging bravery rather than permitting avoidance in each of those seven areas. For example, it is better to teach someone to participate in group activities—even in small and gradual doses—than to allow him to avoid them. Avoidance of team or group interaction such as turn taking, listening, and allowing others to lead will most likely serve to increase a person's belief that he is unsure how to participate and can simply follow his own ideas and choices without listening to the ideas of others. Similarly, the more we allow a student or client to avoid the school playground, the more likely he is to feel that he does not know how to initiate or sustain play with his peers. Furthermore, we might also be isolating him from his peers. This can reinforce any possible thoughts that his peers have that there is something "wrong with" or "weird" about the student or client.

Ultimately, if you want to help reduce anxiety in your student or client, then you will need to be prepared to experience short-term challenges in his behavior. You will need to allow him to make mistakes, and to experience anxiety so that he can learn that the object of his fear is perhaps not actually as bad as he believes it to be. Perhaps you will also need to allow yourself to experience worry and anxiety to learn that you are more capable of assisting him than you might have initially thought.

Strategies for Working with an Anxious Student or Client with Autism

Given that encouraging bravery seems to be the better of the two options we've presented, what are the specific techniques and strategies an education or healthcare professional can use to do this? Below are twelve strategies or "indirect treatments" to help professionals reduce anxiety and increase coping, independence, and self-confidence in their student or client. Several of the strategies below are similar to what was discussed for parents in Chapter 5. However, clearly the application of them in a classroom or clinic is quite different from what it might be in a family setting. Therefore, included are some examples of how you might apply each strategy within your classroom or clinical setting. Please note that these are simply suggestions. After reading them, you will probably be able to generate a personalized list of techniques and examples for your own students or clients.

1. Praise Brave Behavior

Frequently noticing the efforts of your students or clients being brave pays dividends for all concerned. Making such a concerted effort to praise them specifically for brave behavior requires that you pay closer attention to even small examples of brave, confident, or independent behavior. It is important that the language you use clearly highlights to the person that you have picked up on the details of his efforts to be brave. Praising someone for his bravery helps him become more aware himself of *exactly* what it is about his behavior that shows less fear and more confidence. On that basis, he is more likely to understand how to try to display this behavior again. If you are an education or healthcare professional working with an anxious person with autism, then I strongly recommend that you write up your own list of phrases or praising statements like those listed below. Refer to your written list as often as possible (e.g., daily if you are the classroom teacher). From the examples below, you can also see that you do not need to wait for the students or clients to totally overcome their fears in order to praise them for bravery. In fact, if you start by finding small examples of confidence and bravery, then you'll probably find that you are able to praise them more often than if you are waiting for something "big" to happen. Some examples of praise for students or clients include:

- *"Congratulations on being so brave and starting your handwriting sheet without my help!"*
- *"I am so proud of you for speaking up with a nice clear voice during circle time/sharing today. You were so confident when you talked to the other children about your cousin's new house."*

- *"It was amazing to watch you leave Mom right away when I called you into my office and to see the brave expression on your face."*
- *"I can see that you are really trying to get through your assignments more on your own without checking with the other students to see whether or not you are on the right track. It's a pleasure to see that kind of self-confidence growing in you."*
- *"You've been putting a huge amount of effort into completing your practice tasks for me without worrying about making a mistake. That tells me you are really getting the hang of being brave and giving it a go. Good for you!"*

Typically, for students with higher support needs you might need to use a visual cue such as a picture of a brave face to accompany simpler statements such as:

- *"You've been staying calm throughout the whole lesson. Great job!"*
- *"You've been brave during the noisy music class. Awesome!"*

2. Pay Close Attention to Brave Behavior and Independence

Spending extra time with students or clients with autism when they are showing independence or bravery is another way that we can positively reinforce their behavior. We can show our attention through our own behavior including smiles, simple affection, sitting alongside them and watching them eagerly, giving a concrete reward like class table points, a sticker, or a pick from the classroom goody bag, or engaging in silly or over-the-top behavior like dancing on the spot or doing jumping jacks to celebrate their bravery. Over-the-top behavior is a great response for a professional to use. Students or clients rarely expect you to engage in silly behavior in front of them, especially in celebration of a brave or confident act. Catching them by surprise in this way is a very salient way to let them know just how pleased you are to see their efforts to be brave. Below are some examples of how to pay closer attention to brave behavior:

- Walking over to a child when he is completing work independently (e.g., a math worksheet), then stopping him briefly so that you can give him a big smile or pat on the back as you tell him how proud of him you are for being brave and doing the task on his own.

- Stating something like, "I noticed that you just chose your book for reading practice on your own. I'd love to sit beside you and listen to you read because I can see how confidently you are getting ready and I love to watch you when you are being confident with your reading."
- Doing jumping jacks in response to seeing that a student has listened and coped when you have announced a change in the routine.
- Pretending to be a TV news announcer and announcing a news flash to the whole class or clinic group about the child's bravery in coping.
- Giving a student or client a special reward (e.g., five to ten minutes of computer time, one hundred extra table points, or perhaps even a special bravery ribbon that you have made) to encourage him when he has given a presentation in front of a group of his peers.

When using verbal attention like praise and nonverbal attention like affection, time, and over-the-top behavior, it is critical that you always respond **immediately**, that is, as soon as you notice the bravery or confidence. All people—whether or not they have autism—benefit from instant, positive reinforcement for their brave behavior rather than a response that comes later in the day. Delayed responses make it harder for a person to realize that what you are saying or doing is a direct result of something brave in his behavior. Consequently, it is harder for him to know to repeat the same brave behavior again next time. So, please *avoid* rewards and phrases such as, "Because you were so brave in staying with the class for the morning assembly, we'll let you choose which book the whole class can read during our reading circle time tomorrow."

If the person does not seem to like being the center of attention, then you needn't single him out in front of his peers. For example, walking over and whispering praise to a student can be just as rewarding as announcing it in front of the class. To be equitable in a classroom setting, it is also a good idea to pay attention to other students' bravery and praise them too. In this way, the student with autism does not feel singled out and the other students get equal treatment.

3. Set Goals

Often people become easily overwhelmed when they are anxious, thinking that their fears are insurmountable. When we are trying to conquer fears or worries, it is always best to break the worries down into smaller, more realistic and achievable steps. We are better off setting small goals that we can work on a step at a time. Then, once we have conquered a small goal, we feel more confident and less overwhelmed moving to a more challenging task. Below is an example of how you might break down a handwriting activity into small steps for an elementary school student with anxiety about this particular task:

Goal Breakdown for Overcoming Anxiety about Handwriting

- Goal/Step 1: Trace over one word.
- Goal/Step 2: Trace over half a sentence.
- Goal/Step 3: Trace over a full sentence.
- Goal/Step 4: Free-hand writing of individual letters.
- Goal/Step 5: Free-hand writing of single words.
- Goal/Step 6: Free-hand writing of half a sentence.
- Goal/Step 7: Free-hand writing of a full sentence.
- Goal/Step 8: Free-hand writing of two sentences.
- Goal/Step 9: Free-hand writing of a paragraph.
- Goal/Step 10: Free-hand writing of one page from a favorite book.

The following example demonstrates how to break down a worry of an elementary school student about speaking in front of the class:

Goal Breakdown for Overcoming a Fear of Public Speaking

- Goal/Step 1: Answer a question when asked by the teacher.
- Goal/Step 2: Spontaneously offer to answer a question in front of the class.
- Goal/Step 3: Ask a child a question during "morning news" time.
- Goal/Step 4: Ask the teacher one question in front of the class.

- Goal/Step 5: Ask the teacher two questions in front of the class.
- Goal/Step 6: Read aloud during reading groups.
- Goal/Step 7: Have a conversation with the teacher in front of the class (e.g., during "circle time").
- Goal/Step 8: Give news.
- Goal/Step 9: Give a presentation about yourself for "Star of the Week."
- Goal/Step 10: Lead a small group project.

It is important that we set realistic goals and start with the goal or step that seems most manageable or easiest to achieve. Again, we want to set the person up to succeed, so going straight to Step 10 on the list above would not lead to success. The more the student practices each step or works towards each goal, the more likely he is to feel comfortable in doing the feared activity.

4. Proportional Rewards

For each of the steps or goals that are set and conquered, it is vital that the child be rewarded. Rewards are not bribes. A bribe is what we might give someone when we want him to do something that is of benefit to us; but a reward is what we give to a person who has put effort into achieving something for himself. When choosing rewards for anxious individuals, it is important that they are proportional to the task. In other words, rewards need to match the level of difficulty or anxiety associated with the goal or challenge that is set. Going back to the example earlier of the steps in overcoming a fear of handwriting, we might allocate smaller level rewards such as praise or doing "the wave" with the class for smaller steps (e.g., Steps 1-3). Then we might allocate a big reward such as extra time on the computer for more challenging steps (e.g., Steps 4-7). Finally, we would give the biggest reward such as choosing a toy from a goody box, a gift certificate to a preferred store, or a special award or certificate and prize for the most challenging steps (e.g., Steps 8-10). Naturally, it is important that rewards are age-appropriate and not perceived as embarrassing, especially for teenagers. Therefore, the overall plan for goals toward overcoming a fear of handwriting and the related rewards might look like Table 7.

Table 7	Sample Steps and Rewards Towards Conquering a Fear of Handwriting	
Conquering a fear of handwriting		
Goal/Step	**Reward**	
1. Trace over one word	Praise and a special handshake or high-five	
2. Trace over half a sentence	Jumping jacks from the teacher or healthcare professional	
3. Trace over a full sentence	"The wave" in the classroom or clinic	
4. Free-hand writing of individual letters	Extra table points for your class table	
5. Free-hand writing of single words	Picking the order of activities to be completed in the class or clinic that day	
6. Free-hand writing of half a sentence	Extra time on the class computer or on the healthcare professional's computer	
7. Free-hand writing of a full sentence	Time playing a board game	
8. Free-hand writing of two sentences	Picking a small treat from a goody bag	
9. Free-hand writing of a paragraph	Gift certificate to a preferred store	
10. Free-hand writing of one page from a favorite book	Being given a school principal's or clinic award/certificate and prize	

Again, it is helpful to remember that rewards need to be delivered immediately, that is, as soon as the person carries out the set task. It is also important to remember that rewards need to be given every time the person carries out the set task. Therefore, if a child was to practice Step 1 three times in a week, then he would also be given praise and a special handshake in immediate response three times that week.

5. Planned Ignoring of Non-brave Behavior

As stated earlier, we need to give more attention to brave behavior and less attention to non-brave behavior. Giving less attention to non-brave behavior can involve a technique called "planned ignoring." Essentially, we briefly acknowledge that the person might feel worried or anxious but then we try to move away from him once we have given a suggestion regarding what he can do to cope better. It is important that we are able to ignore someone when he becomes anxious or fearful rather than respond to behaviors such as repetitive questioning, checking, fretting, or avoidance. We need to show the anxious individual that we will give plenty of attention and reinforcement when he is brave; not when he is anxious. It is not harsh or cruel to remove attention when a person is showing an unhelpful level of worry or anxiety. Rather, it is better for him to learn that he is much better spending his energy being brave because less time and attention is given to him when he is not coping. Remember, the objects or situations that most of us fear, including those of who have autism, are usually innocuous or safe. Therefore:

- Avoid answering a child every time he repeatedly asks you to go through the daily school or clinic session routine to ensure that there are no changes to what he predicts is the correct order of activities or tasks.
- Avoid complying when a person with autism asks you to rearrange the objects on your office desk so that they are in the same order as they were when he last saw them.
- Limit reassurance and comfort when a child is having a tantrum because he lost a board game or was unable to line up first when you asked the class to get ready to go outside for recess.
- Avoid or limit conversation with an adolescent when he wants to discuss all the reasons why he doesn't want to participate in a group research activity with his classmates.
- Limit time spent trying to reason and reassure a teenager with autism who seems anxious about starting conversations with other people his age when you have agreed to set this as a social skills homework task.

6. Model Brave Behavior

We can develop bravery and confidence in others by modeling that kind of behavior for them. The more we display bravery and confidence in our own actions, the more other people are likely to pick up on this style of behavior as a better way to approach their own fears or worries. Education and healthcare professionals who work with people with autism, more often than not, are able to establish good relationships with their students or clients. They are respected and seen as good role models. Hence, if an education or healthcare professional were to deliberately display more confident or brave behavior in front of a student or client, then that student or client might pay more attention to his own brave behavior. Often, it is helpful to narrate, or talk through our brave behavior as we display it. We can also over-demonstrate or over-dramatize it so that it is very clear. For example:

- *"I'm scared that I won't get my report done on time for a family I am working with. I'll just keep telling myself that everything will be alright. I've never handed a report in late before and if I do, it's not the end of the world."*

- *"I can't seem to get my worried thoughts out of my head about all of the work I have to finish. Maybe I should try to distract myself whenever I feel like that. I could try to think about what I'm most looking forward to about my weekend to help clear away my worried thoughts."*

- *"I really don't like the taste of mango. It feels gross in my mouth. But I'm going to be brave today and try a small piece of it with some yogurt so that I can start to get used to it. After all, just because something doesn't taste very good, doesn't mean it's bad for you. If I keep trying it, I might get used to it."*

- *"I heard this morning that it might rain early next week. I'm worried that the campout might be cancelled. I probably just need to keep reminding myself that, even if it is cancelled, we can go another time."*

- *"I feel a little distracted today because my son is at home with the flu and his dad is taking care of him. I need to be confident and tell myself that he's going to get better soon and he's in good hands."*

Just as would be helpful for parents at home, video modeling might be a useful adjunct to the above suggestions for professionals. You could video record your own examples of brave behavior and then play these back to help "coach" your student or client regarding how to approach a situation that he is afraid of. Similarly, it might be both a helpful and a fun exercise for younger children with autism to try to spot examples of brave behavior in cartoon characters, actors/actresses, or other celebrities that they relate to. As noted above, when we see people we admire engaging in brave behavior, we are likely to try to emulate them.

What is Video Modeling?

Video modeling is a mode of teaching that uses video recording and playback to provide a visual model of the behavior or skill that you're trying to teach. Using video modeling, the child learns by observation. Desired behaviors are video recorded and then played back to the person so that he can watch exactly what is involved in exhibiting a behavior. The video footage can be used to "coach" the person regarding exactly what to say, how to look, and what gestures to use. By playing and re-playing the video footage for the "correct" behavior, the person is better able to learn what is required of him and display the same behavior.

---

7. Role Reversal

We all know that children and adolescents like to have a turn at telling an adult what to do. Role reversal allows them to do this with a special focus on teaching an adult how to be more brave and confident. By coaching you in what to do when you feel worried (even if you rarely feel worried and do not need this kind of coaching), the person with autism is more likely to adopt the same advice. Consider some of the following ideas that you might use with children or adolescents:

For a child…"I'm not sure how to stop myself from thinking about my meeting tomorrow and talking in front of all those people. You're usually really good at being brave. Can you teach me what to do so that I can feel brave?"

For a child…"I saw another cockroach in my house last night. I felt so worried that it would crawl near my foot and leave germs in my house. I've seen you taking some big breaths when you feel scared. Can you show me what you do? I think it might help me feel more confident next time I see a cockroach in my house."

For an adolescent…"I noticed that you were really confident when you presented that research in front of the class this afternoon. I've got a staff presentation that I'm preparing for and I'm feeling overwhelmed about it. What did you do today to help you stay so confident when you spoke? Can you show me? I think it might work for me too."

For an adolescent…"I've got so much grading to do from the exam and I just don't seem to feel confident that it will all get done. You're very good at staying calm when you have lots of school work and assignments to get through. What do you tell yourself to help you get it done? Maybe it will work for me too."

The key with role reversal is asking for help so that you take on the apprentice role in order to boost the child or adolescent's confidence and sense of competence regarding ways to be brave. It is important to sound sincere toward the person so as to convince him that you really need his advice, so it's doesn't come off as patronizing. Just as was discussed for rewarding brave behavior, it is important that you put effort into finding or creating opportunities for the child or adolescent to coach you. You might not truly believe that he is the best person to tell you or teach you how to be confident. You may even be one of those lucky people who are usually quite confident and rarely worried or anxious. Regardless, you will be pleasantly surprised how young people can rise to the occasion when they feel they are in charge of an adult. They then put more emphasis on displaying brave behavior as an example for you.

8. Allocate Responsibilities and Encourage Independence

As discussed above, it is important to focus attention on bravery not fear. By encouraging a person with autism to "go for it" or take on a task alone, we can help him learn that he can do it and does not always need to rely on adult support to feel comfortable or safe. The best way to foster independence is to find or create opportunities where the person can take on an extra job or responsibility that he completes alone. It does not matter how simple the task is. What matters most is that you reinforce and praise the fact that the person has shown bravery or confidence in completing the task, without assistance. Some examples of key areas that might be targeted for your students or clients are outlined below. Again, it is my hope that from the examples below you might generate a more personalized list of other areas of responsibility to give to your own students or clients:

- Asking a young child to be in charge of putting away a selection of toys on his own in his daycare or preschool.
- Asking a child to be in charge of one area of the classroom, e.g., keeping the computer area uncluttered or monitoring the classroom ant farm.
- Asking a child to be in charge of putting all the reading group books in order each Wednesday to help you stay organized and get all the groups doing their reading tasks quickly.
- Asking an adolescent to become a peer tutor for another student or group of students in an area where the adolescent seems to have more skill or knowledge than his peers.
- Asking an adolescent to take on the role as the school audio/visual (AV) consultant and assist in setting up the AV system for school assemblies or productions.

For people with higher support needs, simpler tasks might work better, for example:

- Asking a child to be in charge of holding the door open as the class files in and out of the classroom.
- Asking a person to be in charge of counting all the class members when lining up outside the classroom.
- Asking a person to be in charge of watering the office plants.

From the examples above, you can see that the tasks are usually just daily, routine activities that the child or adolescent is probably quite capable of doing without any feelings of anxiety. The goal is to identify easy tasks that the person feels comfortable trying unassisted. Consequently, there will be ample opportunities to reward or encourage his confidence or independence in doing them. Again, it is critical that when you see the tasks being completed independently, you praise the person for his confidence, independence, bravery, or effort in doing so without anyone's help. Essentially, we want to set him up to succeed. If you choose tasks where you do not currently see confidence and independence, then you will have a much harder job of finding opportunities to reward bravery. Remember, if you can start with frequently rewarding an individual with autism for his bravery in the simplest of tasks, then he is more likely to apply himself independently to tasks that are genuinely challenging or fear provoking. Also, when a person sees that he is able to take on more tasks independently, he is more likely to feel better about himself—to have higher self-esteem.

It is helpful to "up the ante" regarding the type of tasks you assume the person with anxiety can handle on his own over time. You can judge this by how consistently he is able to complete a task independently. For example, if a student with high support needs can consistently water the office plants over several weeks, then it's time to "raise the bar" by asking him to also be in charge of delivering mail from the office to his teachers.

9. Deliberately Create Opportunities for Change in Their Routine or Environment

It is commonly noted that people with autism have a preference for sameness in their personal and broader environment (e.g., Mesibov, Adams & Klinger, 1997). Consequently, they can become worried or anxious when there is some kind of change. For example, changes in daily routines, their bedroom, their home, their school uniform, their own appearance, or other people's appearance might cause concern for them because of the lack of familiarity.

Much of the literature on supporting individuals with autism identifies the need to prepare or forewarn them of changes. For example, visual schedules are often suggested as a means of explaining the daily routine and highlighting clearly when and how a change might occur. However, often professionals ask me whether it is better to allow changes in their students' or clients' routines or environment or to keep the routines and environment as consistent as possible in order to avoid any anxiety that might arise. If we consider the question of change as another example of facing fears and encouraging bravery then, in general, the answer would be to encourage change; indeed, to create more opportunities for change so that the person becomes more and more used to it in his routines and environment. Some examples might include:

- Regularly changing the way the books in the reading corner of the classroom are arranged.

- Regularly changing the location of toys in your office.
- Regularly changing the order of classroom activities (e.g., reading before math groups instead of after writing).
- Regularly changing the look of your classroom bulletin boards.
- Regularly changing the seating positions within the classroom.
- Regularly changing the order of the activities you complete in a therapy session.

As suggested in much of the scientific literature, change will be best introduced by forewarning the person of the change but ignoring any of the protests. It is helpful to start with smaller, less significant changes then move to more significant ones as the person begins to show more resilience. Again, it is essential to couple changes in routines or the environment with rewards and praise for bravery whenever the person shows coping behavior.

10. Restructure Tasks

Often people with autism become easily overwhelmed by learning tasks. It can be during these moments of feeling overwhelmed when we observe challenging behavior such as task refusal, negotiating or bargaining a way out of the task, yelling, or tantrums. Like most of us, when a person with autism is overwhelmed by a task, it is often because he cannot clearly see a way to navigate through the task. That is, the task seems daunting because he cannot see how the task can be broken down into smaller steps to complete one at a time.

The use of interactive, visual work systems (e.g., as outlined in the evidence-based TEACCH approach to visual support for individuals with autism; Mesibov, Shea & Schopler, 2005) is a key way for education professionals, especially, to help students overcome any anxiety they feel about starting or completing a learning task. By breaking a learning task down into smaller, less anxiety-provoking steps and providing a system to help the person track his own progress through the task, then you can reduce the student's anxiety and help him complete work more independently. The use of activity schedules can also help people feel more "in control" and less anxious about work by allowing them to better understand what to expect as they move through their day.

In using work systems to manage task anxiety, it is critical that you are able to visually show the student the answers to some key questions:

- What is the work?
- How much work is there?
- How do I make progress through the work?
- What happens next, i.e., when the work is finished?

Consider the example of a math worksheet (Figure 2 helps to highlight this point). A student might receive the worksheet and instantly become anxious thinking about the fact that he struggles with math and, therefore, does not want to complete the task. However, if he is able to see visually on the worksheet that, rather than a page of calculations, it's actually broken down into several numbered sections, with boxes to check off as he completes each section, and clear instructions at the end of the worksheet regarding what to do when he finishes, then the student might be more likely to get started on the task without protest. Even though the second worksheet might look as though it contains more work than the original, it helps the student see the breakdown of the required calculations into sections that can be completed one at a time and is, therefore, likely to seem less overwhelming.

Figure 3 helps illustrate how you might change an English comprehension activity into a task that is less intimidating for a person with autism and anxiety. It also ensures that the steps involved are clear and easy to follow.

Essentially, the point of a work system is to allow people to work independently but in a way that is better structured so that they feel less overwhelmed and more motivated to remain on task (Mesibov, Shea & Schopler, 2005).

If you think about it, we all use work systems to help reduce our own sense of feeling overwhelmed or pressured. For example, every day when I enter the clinic and on my desk is a pile of work to be completed, I write a list of all the tasks I need to finish. Then, I prioritize the list, stack the tasks on the left side of my desk in order and, as each task is completed, I place it in the finished tray on the right side of my desk. It gives me great satisfaction as I cross off each completed task on my list. The receptionist uses a similar system with the "In/Out" trays and memo pads on his desk. There are many other examples of how we use work systems in our daily lives to help us remain organized and, in turn, reduce feelings of anxiety or pressure. Therefore, it makes sense that people with autism would benefit from seeing how to complete a challenging learning task in a way that breaks the task down into manageable steps.

Figure 2 | Sample of a Restructured Math Worksheet

Original Math Worksheet

Write your answers in the spaces below:

1. $4 + 7 =$ _____
2. $10 - 3 =$ _____
3. $8 + 1 - 2 =$ _____
4. $3 + 8 - 5 =$ _____
5. $12 + 7 =$ _____
6. $19 + 1 =$ _____

Restructured Math Worksheet

Write your answers in the spaces below:
Place a check mark (✓) in the box (□) after you finish each section:

Section 1:

$4 + 7 =$ _____
$10 - 3 =$ _____

□ Place a check mark (✓) in the box (□) after you have finished Section 1.

Section 2:

$8 + 1 - 2 =$ _____
$3 + 8 - 5 =$ _____

□ Place a check mark (✓) in the box (□) after you have finished Section 2.

Section 3:

$12 + 7 =$ _____
$19 + 1 =$ _____

□ Place a check mark (✓) in the box (□) after you have finished Section 3.

FINISHED! WELL DONE!
Put your worksheet into your math exercise binder.

Figure 3 | Sample of a Restructured English Worksheet

Original English Task

Write about the main characters in the book. What are their strengths and weaknesses?

_____

_____

_____

_____

_____

_____

_____

Restructured English Task

Place a check mark (✓) in the box (☐) after you finish each section:

1. Write the names of the two main characters in the book?   ☐

Character's Name: _____

Character's Name _____

2. List three strengths and three weaknesses for each character.   ☐

Character's Name	Strengths	Weaknesses
_____	1. _____	1. _____
	2. _____	2. _____
	3. _____	3. _____
Character's Name	Strengths	Weaknesses
_____	1. _____	1. _____
	2. _____	2. _____
	3. _____	3. _____

(continued on next page)

3. Use the words in your lists to write three sentences about each character's strengths and weaknesses. ☐

Character's Name: _____

Sentences about their strengths:

   1. _____

   2. _____

   3. _____

Sentences about their weaknesses:

   1. _____

   2. _____

   3. _____

Character's Name: _____

Sentences about their strengths:

   1. _____

   2. _____

   3. _____

Sentences about their weaknesses:

   1. _____

   2. _____

   3. _____

4. Check your spelling and punctuation. ☐

FINISHED!
Put your worksheet on the teacher's desk.

11. Sensory Desensitization

Often the school years are particularly challenging for children with autism because of the sensory sensitivities they have. Many kids find that playgrounds and other areas where large groups of students gather are too noisy or too visually stimulating. Similarly, others might have difficulty with tactile sensitivities, finding particular aspects of their school clothes or uniform uncomfortable to wear. Their tactile sensitivities might also make other activities like art difficult to participate in. People with sensory sensitivities may experience anxiety when asked to attend school assemblies, go onto the playground, participate in a music or art lesson, or maintain their uniform according to school dress codes. Again, it's a good idea for education and healthcare professionals to encourage students and their families to gradually expose and desensitize people with autism to their feared sensory experience(s) rather than avoid them completely. Examples might include:

- encouraging gradually longer attendance during school assemblies;
- encouraging gradually longer periods of time on the school playground;
- encouraging gradual participation in tactile experiences like arts and crafts, e.g., at first simply using a paintbrush, then perhaps fingerpainting, then touching glue, then exploring other mediums; and
- encouraging a student to gradually change from wearing t-shirts to wearing long-sleeved shirts as the weather gets colder.

You can use praise or other forms of reward to encourage your students or clients to do the types of things listed in the examples above. The previous sections on setting goals (#3) and using proportional rewards (#4) contain more ideas to help you do this.

12. Incorporate Intense or Unusual Interests into the Curriculum

As discussed above, sometimes students with autism feel easily overwhelmed by learning tasks because of their language and communication difficulties. To assist in reducing anxiety at these times, it is recommended that education professionals consider ways to incorporate students' interests into the curriculum. Doing so helps ensure students are more motivated to try assignments. Consequently, they are more easily rewarded and reinforced for being brave and attempting a work task. Some examples from my own clients include:

- When a student was anxious about literacy tasks but had a special interest in cars, then attempts were made to allow him to read books about cars or write short passages about "Top Gear," his preferred TV show.

- When a student was worried about completing math tasks but had a special interest in garbage cans, then attempts were made to write unique math problems for the student that focused on calculations regarding trash, garbage cans, garbage truck routes, and recycling. For example: Calculate the time it will take a garbage truck to travel five miles from the depot to the first house on its route if it is travelling an average speed of twenty-five miles per hour.

- When a student was overwhelmed by the thought of giving presentations in front of the class but had a special interest in football, then attempts were made to allow the student to present a weekly sports report to the class including a rundown of the week's football game results.

Sometimes classroom teachers are understandably concerned about the idea of preparing separate work for a student with special needs, especially in a mainstream setting. They might think that it is unfair to allow one student to complete work regarding his own interests when other students are not given the same opportunity. However, the aim of incorporating a student's interests in his curriculum is to ultimately help him complete learning tasks that are the same as those of his peers.

The students in the examples above could see that they were able to complete some of the tasks they feared when their special interests were incorporated. Consequently, they were more confident about extending themselves to completing the same activities as their classmates without including their special interests. The point to emphasize again is that in order to instill confidence in students with autism, it is important to try to set them up to succeed. In other words, we first need to provide opportunities for them to see that they are capable of completing the task at all before we can start setting firmer boundaries around them doing the same work as their fellow students. The most obvious way to ensure this is to use their interests to better engage and motivate them in their learning.

In Summary

- As professionals, we are presented with a dilemma regarding how best to support an anxious student or client with autism: Do we encourage him to be brave and face his fears or do we permit avoidance of the feared object or situation?
- Sometimes professionals can themselves become anxious regarding working with students with autism because of some misconceptions including:
  - All people with autism present with challenging behavior.
  - Autism is an area for specialists or requires "new" approaches. Therefore, I do not have enough skills or experience to help.
  - Supporting a child with autism will involve too much extra work.
  - It's not fair to the other students to give individual assistance to a student with autism.
- Education and healthcare professionals usually have a wealth of experience and skills to assist people with autism. Often they do not need "new" or specialty approaches but rather to call on long-standing, scientifically-supported strategies that have been applied for decades to other groups of people and are equally beneficial to people with autism.
- It is healthier for professionals to encourage bravery in their students or clients with autism than to encourage them to avoid what they fear. The more we support people avoiding a fear, the more anxious they will become.
- Avoidance increases anxiety because it limits the number of opportunities an individual has to face the feared

object or situation and learn that he can probably cope if he remains in the situation for long enough.

- Teachers and healthcare professionals can help reduce anxiety and boost self-confidence in their students or clients by:
  - ❑ Praising bravery
  - ❑ Giving extra attention to brave or independent behavior
  - ❑ Setting goals
  - ❑ Giving proportional rewards
  - ❑ Ignoring non-brave behavior
  - ❑ Modeling brave behavior
  - ❑ Role reversal
  - ❑ Allocating responsibilities
  - ❑ Deliberately creating opportunities for change in their routine or environment
  - ❑ Restructuring tasks
  - ❑ Sensory desensitization
  - ❑ Incorporating intense or unusual interests into the curriculum

Part III

Direct Treatments for Anxiety

7 | **Direct Treatments for Anxiety: Psychoanalytic Treatment, Alternative Medicine, and Medication**

Tim and the Rossen Family

Tim has a diagnosis of autism and is a high functioning eighth grader in an inclusive setting. Tim's parents contact me sporadically when they have questions regarding Tim's management. Recently, they came to see me about his anxiety difficulties. They told me that since starting eighth grade, Tim's anxiety has grown the more aware he becomes of his upcoming transition to high school next year. The Rossens note that Tim worries about being able to cope with the workload, the change in structure, the different subject teachers, and the large number of students. He also worries particularly about how he will manage to make friends. Mr. and Mrs. Rossen discussed that Tim's anxiety seems to have reached a head in the past three weeks. Apparently, many times throughout the day, Tim worries about transitioning to high school and seems unable to concentrate on other activities. They told me that Tim also seems to be losing sleep because of worry and is not eating as much as he usually does. He has lost weight and is experiencing regular bouts of diarrhea.

Mrs. Rossen told me that, before coming to see me, she had gone online and read about anxiety treatments. Having found a range of sites suggesting a range of treatment options, what Mrs. Rossen wanted was my advice on which treatment approach would be best for Tim. Was medication the best approach? Should they put him onto fish oil supplements? Should they take him to see a psychiatrist? What does psychodynamic therapy mean? Both parents seemed extremely confused. Of course, as *many parents would, they had also sought opinions from several other parents within a support group they attend. Naturally, each parent they spoke to had their own opinions about what form of treatment might be best. Unfortunately, the wide range of opinions only added to Tim's parents' confusion.*

The Rossens are not the first set of parents who have come to me asking about the best treatment approach for their anxious child. There are many options available to families and it is not always clear which one is best. As a clinical psychologist, my training and the evidence I read suggests that Cognitive Behavioral intervention (CBT) is a good approach to treating anxiety difficulties in people with autism. CBT will be discussed in much more detail in Chapter 8. However, there are several other treatment approaches that exist and deserve further discussion.

I want to be especially clear that I am by no means an expert on all of the various forms of anxiety treatments that exist for people with autism. Therefore, in this chapter my aim is not to tell you what to believe or what treatment approach to follow; rather, I simply want to outline some of the key intervention approaches that do exist, along with any scientific support or concerns that might surround them. I intend to give you some brief information regarding what each treatment targets, what is involved, and any evidence that exists in the scientific literature regarding how effective the treatment is. The decision as to whether or not the treatments described herein are suitable for your child, family, student, or client is yours to make.

Despite the strong evidence that anxiety difficulties occur commonly in people with autism and result in marked distress to families, there has been little research into effective treatment options. Cognitive behavior therapy (CBT) will be discussed at length in Chapter 8 as one treatment option that we have begun to use. However, before CBT began to be applied to people with autism, the two main forms of intervention were psychoanalytic treatment (used more frequently in the past) and medication (or pharmacotherapy). There has also been some use of other more alternative therapies/counseling strategies and alternative medicine such as the use of vitamins and supplements. We will focus on psychoanalytic treatments, alternative therapies, alternative medicine, and medication briefly in this chapter with the strongest focus on medication, as it seems to be the most commonly adopted form of treatment for anxiety.

Psychoanalytic Treatment

In general, psychoanalytic treatments emphasize resolving unconscious mental conflicts. Therefore, treatments have focused on three areas of "conflict" for people with autism (Braconnier, 1983; Heinemann, 1999; Schteingart, 1989):

- Exploring the client's "separation anxiety" from her therapist.
- Exploring anxiety relating to a disturbance in the "primary bond" between the client and her mother.
- Exploring the client's "body anxiety" in order to help the client address the physiological component of her anxiety response.

In the past, some researchers argued that individuals who underwent counseling or "analysis" using a psychoanalytic approach made gains in terms of reduced anxiety and reduced physiological symptoms such as reduced panic. However, when exploring the research regarding psychoanalytic treatments for anxiety in autism, there seem to be three key limitations. First, the extent of the scientific research that supported the use of psychoanalytic therapy was limited. Most of the studies that explored the efficacy of psychoanalytic techniques involved very small numbers of people, indeed, often only one person. Therefore, there is probably not enough evidence to suggest that psychoanalysis should be the treatment of choice if we do not have information regarding the benefits of this kind of approach for large numbers of anxious people with autism.

Second, there is little information about measurable change for people from before their treatment to after completing their treatment. In other words, there was no standardized measurement of change in anxiety symptoms for the participants in the research. When there is no standardized or systematic measurement of change in symptoms, then it is hard to know whether what I might consider to be reduction in anxiety is the same as what another clinician might consider a reduction in anxiety. Consequently, beyond a clinician's subjective opinion, we cannot easily determine whether people with autism who received psychoanalytic therapy actually showed any improvements by the end of their treatment.

Third, the psychoanalytic techniques employed in research studies, including exploring anxiety relating to a disturbance in the primary bond between the client and her mother, seemed to be based on the premise that the quality of child-parent relationships is a cause of autism. This notion was otherwise referred to in early scientific literature by Beetelheim as "refrigerator parent" syndrome (Wing, 1997). Theories suggesting that one of the causes of autism is a "refrigerator mother" (a parent who is emotionally distant from her child) have been discredited in scientific literature (Wing, 1997). Therefore, any treatment approaches based on this theory are also difficult to justify.

Alternative Therapies

Naturally, there are a host of more alternative style therapies/counseling approaches that families might access to address anxiety difficulties in their son or daughter with an ASD. Techniques and therapies include but are not limited to:

- art therapy
- dance therapy
- drama therapy
- Eye Movement Desensitization and Reprocessing (EMDR)
- family therapy
- music therapy
- narrative therapy
- play therapy
- supportive counseling

Currently, it is not possible to make an evidence-based judgment about the effectiveness of these approaches because of lack of scientific literature regarding their use in treating anxiety in people with an ASD. While each therapeutic approach might have merit in treating a range of mental health issues, I am somewhat skeptical about their ability to directly target the core symptoms of anxiety discussed in Chapter 1. Therefore, until a body of evidence is established that supports the use of such treatments for anxiety in people with an ASD, I would not recommend families seek out such interventions to address anxiety in their son or daughter with autism.

Alternative Medicine

The use of complementary and alternative medicine (CAM) for people with autism seems to have gathered support and momentum in the past few years. Surveys have indicated that up to 74 percent of families have explored complementary medicine for their child with autism (e.g., Hanson, Kalish, Bunce, Curtis, McDaniel, Ware & Petry, 2007). Complementary and alternative approaches include:

- Special diets (e.g., gluten-free, casein-free, wheat-free, sugar-free, dairy-free)
- Inclusion of extra vitamins or minerals (e.g., Vitamin B6 and Magnesium)
- Food supplements (e.g., omega-3 fatty acids and fish oil)
- Herbal remedies (e.g., Passiflora, St. John's Wort, Chamomile)
- Massage and/or body-work therapies (e.g., chiropractic and osteopathic manipulation, acupuncture)

Interestingly, the parents surveyed did not necessarily explore complementary and alternative medicine to specifically target anxiety difficulties in their child; rather, they seemed to make use of these treatments as a means of addressing the core difficulties in social skills, communication, and behavior, with the possibility that there might be indirect benefits such as reduced anxiety.

A review of the literature indicates only one study that has used complementary and alternative medicine to directly target anxiety in an individual with an ASD. Johnson and Hollander (2003) used fish oil supplements with omega-3 fatty acids (1g to 3g daily) to assist in reducing anxiety in an eleven-year-old boy with autism. They reported significant reductions in the boy's anxiety difficulties and his levels of agitation. However, it is important to note that the fish oil supplements were used in addition to two other forms of treatment: medication and behavioral treatment (Johnson & Hollander, 2003). Therefore, it is difficult to determine whether or not using supplements made a significant difference in reducing the boy's anxiety beyond what might have occurred from the inclusion of the medication and behavioral treatment. How can we tell what part of the reduction in anxiety was related to the inclusion of supplements and what part was related to medication or behavioral treatment?

In general, scientists suggest that research regarding complementary and alternative medicine for people with autism needs to be interpreted with caution. Currently, there is little research clearly supporting the efficacy of complementary and alternative treatments for any aspect of autism, including anxiety difficulties. Of the research that does exist, some concerns have been noted about the quality of the research itself. For example, criticism has been made of the lack of double-blind, controlled clinical trials used to investigate dietary intervention (e.g., Harrison Elder, Shankar, Shuster, Theriaque, Burns & Sherrill, 2006). A double-blind experimental procedure is one in which neither the subjects of the experiment nor the persons administering the experiment know the critical aspects of the experiment such as which treatment they are accessing. Double-blind procedures are used in research to guard against both bias from the experimenters toward achieving certain results that might favor their hypothesis and placebo effects from the participants. If double-blind procedures are not used in studies investigating complementary and alternative medicine for people with an ASD, then it makes it harder to give credence to any suggestions that the alternative approaches really do work. How do we know that the effects are not placebo effects?

Researchers such as Pfeiffer et al. (1995) have listed other methodological shortcomings in studies on complementary and alternative medicine. Criticisms have related to a lack of defining vitamin dosage, small numbers of participants in the studies, and a lack of well-standardized and reliable rating scales to measure any change.

In summary, the use of complementary and alternative approaches to treating anxiety in people with autism is still in its infancy. Perhaps more rigorous research is needed before strong conclusions can be made about whether or not they really work.

Common Medications for Treating Anxiety

A wide range of medications are used to treat anxiety disorders in people with autism, just as they are for the general population. The main types of medication are listed below.

Benzodiazepines (Anti-anxiety Medications)

What Are Common Examples of Benzodiazepines?

The main benzodiazepines used to treat anxiety disorders include:

- Alprazolam (Xanax)
- Clonazepam (Klonopin)
- Diazepam (Valium)

- Oxazepam (Serax)
- Chlordiazepoxide (Librium)

How Do They Work?

Benzodiazepines enhance the effect of a neurotransmitter or brain chemical, called gamma-aminobutyric acid, which results in a sedative and muscle relaxing effect. They are generally considered safe and effective in the short term. Moreover, they are considered "quick-acting," i.e., start working almost right away without needing to build up in the system. However, in the longer term, people can develop a tolerance to benzodiazepines. That is, they might need higher doses to get the same effect. Furthermore, some people might become dependent upon them. Therefore, doctors usually prescribe the medication for short periods. People can also experience withdrawal syndrome if they have been taking benzodiazepines for long periods and then stop.

What Types of Anxiety Do They Target?

(Note: Descriptions of these anxiety disorders can be found in Chapter 1.)
- Panic Disorder
- Social Anxiety Disorder/Social Phobia
- Generalized Anxiety Disorder

What Are the Common Side Effects?
- Drowsiness
- Dizziness
- Reduced alertness and concentration

Antidepressants

How Do They Work?

Antidepressants were developed to treat depression. However, they are also considered beneficial in treating people with anxiety disorders because of the overlap in symptoms between anxiety and depression, e.g., the physiological symptoms and negative thinking patterns discussed in Chapter 1. Anxiety often co-occurs with depression. Indeed, a national comorbidity survey in the US indicated that 51 percent of people who suffer with major depression also experience anxiety. There are three main types of antidepressants used to treat anxiety disorders.

The three types outlined below differ mainly in their chemical structure and, therefore, which neurotransmitters (brain chemicals) they affect:

1. Tricyclic antidepressants
   The main tricyclic antidepressants used to treat anxiety disorders include:
   - Imipramine (Tofranil)
   - Desipramine (Norpramin, Pertofrane, and others)
   - Nortriptyline (Aventyl or Pamelor)
   - Amitriptyline (Elavil)
   - Doxepin (Sinequan or Adapin)
   - Clomipramine (Anafranil)
   - Venlafaxine (Effexor)

2. Monoamine oxidase inhibitors (MAOIs)
   The main MAOIs used to treat anxiety disorders include:
   - Phenelzine (Nardil)
   - Tranylcypromine (Parnate)

3. Selective serotonin reuptake inhibitors (SSRIs)
   The main SSRIs used to treat anxiety disorders include:
   - Fluoxetine (Prozac)
   - Fluvoxamine (Luvox)
   - Sertraline (Zoloft)
   - Paroxetine (Paxil)

In general, when treating anxiety disorders, antidepressants are started at low doses and increased slowly over time to help combat any adverse reactions or side effects. Antidepressants tend to take longer to begin relieving anxiety symptoms than the benzodiazepines described above.

It is important to note that people who take MAOIs must avoid certain food (e.g., cheese, bean curd or tofu) and other medications that can interact with this medication and cause dangerous increases in blood pressure.

What Types of Anxiety Do They Target?

(Note: Descriptions of these anxiety disorders can be found in Chapter 1.)

- Panic Disorder
- Generalized Anxiety Disorder
- Obsessive Compulsive Disorder

What Are the Common Side Effects?
- Dry mouth
- Urinary retention
- Blurred vision
- Sedation
- Weight gain
- Headache
- Nausea
- Diarrhea
- Agitation

Beta-blockers

What Are Common Examples of Beta-blockers?
- Propranolol (Inderal)
- Atenolol (Tenormin)

How Do They Work?
Beta-blockers are prescribed to help control some of the physical symptoms of anxiety, such as trembling and sweating. Taking the medicine for a short period of time is suggested to help the person keep physical symptoms under control. However, people can build a tolerance to beta-blockers if they are taken over a long period of time and may need higher and higher doses to get the same effect.

What Types of Anxiety Do They Target?
(Note: Descriptions of these anxiety disorders can be found in Chapter 1.)
Beta-blockers target physical symptoms associated with:
- Social Anxiety Disorder/Social Phobia

What Are the Common Side Effects?
- Increased fatigue
- Cold hands/feet
- Dizziness
- Low blood pressure
- Sudden weight gain

Common Anxiety Disorders and the Medications Often Prescribed for Them

Panic Attacks

Concerning panic attacks, medications are meant to help the patient develop confidence in facing her panic symptoms. In order to do this, medication needs to be helpful in at least one of the two stages of panic. The first stage is anticipatory anxiety, i.e., all the uncomfortable physical symptoms and worries that arise as a person anticipates facing panic. The second stage involves the physical symptoms of the panic attack itself, e.g., racing heart and rapid breathing. Certain medications might help reduce anxiety in either one or in both of these stages. The primary medications used today for Panic Disorder are the benzodiazepines and several types of antidepressants especially the new selective serotonin reuptake inhibitors (SSRIs), sometimes in combination with the benzodiazepines.

Obsessive Compulsive Disorder (OCD)

With regard to obsessions and worries, medications are prescribed to reduce the degree of intensity of the worries and their corresponding distress. Medications do not prevent obsessions or sudden intrusive thoughts from occurring; however, it is argued that, if medication can help reduce the strength of the worry associated with the obsession, then the patient might have a better chance to use other self-help skills to control her obsessions.

Currently, four SSRIs are argued to be helpful in treating OCD: fluoxetine (Prozac), fluvoxamine (Luvox), sertraline (Zoloft), and paroxetine (Paxil). The antidepressants clomipramine (Anafranil) and venlafaxine (Effexor) are also prescribed to assist in treating OCD.

About 20 percent of people with OCD might also have tics. Tics are sudden, uncontrollable physical movements (such as eye blinking) or vocalizations (such as throat clearing). A combination of an SSRI and haloperidol (Haldol) has been used to help such tics and the OCD symptoms.

Generalized Anxiety Disorder (GAD)

In dealing with general anxiety, medications help reduce some of the physical tension symptoms of anxiety. The most commonly prescribed medications for general anxiety are several of the benzodiazepines, such as diazepam (Valium), alprazolam (Xanax), lorazepam (Ativan), oxazepam (Serax), and chlordiazepoxide (Librium). Buspirone (BuSpar) is also used to treat general anxiety.

Social Anxiety Disorder/Social Phobia

When treating social anxieties or phobias, medications can help to reduce the physical tensions or physiological responses associated with entering the feared social situation. That is, they might help to bring a racing heart and sweaty palms under control, and, therefore, to reduce some shyness or insecurity.

The drugs with the longest history of use with social phobias are the beta-blockers. The most commonly used are propranolol (Inderal) and atenolol (Tenormin). However, some research suggests that the monoamine oxidase inhibitors (MAOIs), especially phenelzine, are also effective medications for treating social phobias.

To date, one approach to drug treatment for Social Phobia that some physicians seem to recommend is to take medication only as needed. For example, if patients are anxious only about specific events such as delivering a presentation, then about one hour before the event, they can take certain medications to help reduce their physical anxiety symptoms. However, if the social anxiety goes beyond one or two specific social situations and relates to more general feelings of fear concerning negative evaluation by others across most social situations, then people might be prescribed medication on a daily basis.

Simple Phobias/Specific Phobias

For simple phobias (e.g., fear of heights, flying, snakes), medications might again help to reduce the physical tensions associated with entering the fearful situation. For example, a patient can take a low dose of a benzodiazepine about one hour before facing her feared object or activity to help reduce anticipatory anxiety. If this is not sufficient, then a physician can prescribe a higher dose for the next time.

To simplify, Table 8 on the next page provides a useful summary of the various anxiety disorders and the medications commonly used to treat them.

Table 8	Common Medications Used to Treat Anxiety Disorders	
Type of anxiety disorder	**Type of medication**	**Common medication names**
Panic Disorder	Benzodiazepines	Alprazolam (Xanax) Clonazepam (Klonopin) Diazepam (Valium)
	Antidepressants	Fluoxetine (Prozac) Fluvoxamine (Luvox) Sertraline (Zoloft)
Obsessive Compulsive Disorder (OCD)	Antidepressants	Fluoxetine (Prozac) Fluvoxamine (Luvox) Sertraline (Zoloft) Paroxetine (Paxil) Clomipramine (Anafranil) Venlafaxine (Effexor)
Generalized Anxiety Disorder	Benzodiazepines	Diazepam (Valium) Alprazolam (Xanax) Lorazepam (Ativan) Oxazepam (Serax) Chlordiazepoxide (Librium)
Social Anxiety Disorder/ Social Phobia	Beta-blockers	Propranolol (Inderal) Atenolol (Tenormin)
	Antidepressants	Phenelzine (Nardil)
Simple Phobias/ Specific Phobias	Benzodiazepines	Alprazolam (Xanax) Clonazepam (Klonopin) Diazepam (Valium)

Medication: What Does the Research Say?

Medications such as the selective serotonin reuptake inhibitors (SSRIs) seem to have received the most attention in the treatment literature for anxiety in people with an ASD. Several case studies have explored the benefits of SSRIs in treating anxiety difficulties in people from approximately six years of age through to adolescents. For example, a case report of two children treated with sertraline (daily doses 25 to 50 mg) reported improvements in symptoms of anxiety (Ozbayrak, 1997). However, no objective measures or parent reports were used to assess change in anxiety symptoms. Only clinician observations were reported. Similarly, Bhardwaj et al. (2005) provided a clinical case report of an eleven-year-old girl with an ASD who also had a diagnosis of Separation Anxiety Disorder. After approximately eight weeks of treatment with sertraline (150 mg daily), there was a reported decrease in her anxiety symptoms. However, again, the decrease in anxiety was based solely on clinical observation rather than any standardized assessment measures. Silveira, Jainer and Bates (2004) treated a six-year-old girl, who was diagnosed with Selective Mutism and Social Anxiety Disorder, with fluoxetine (up to 20mg daily). After eight weeks, her parents reported improvements in symptoms of anxiety and Selective Mutism. She was noted as speaking at school and in other environments, and she apparently demonstrated improved eye contact and social smiling.

A larger trial of medication for treating anxiety difficulties in people with an ASD has been conducted with twenty-two youth (twenty with PDD-NOS, two with autism) (Buitelaar et al., 1998). Following six to eight weeks of treatment with buspirone (with doses ranging from 15 to 45 mg daily), sixteen of the individuals showed a positive response: nine had marked improvement and seven had moderate improvement as measured by a standardized improvement scale.

From the above noted results, it seems that medication might help reduce anxiety difficulties in people with an ASD. However, such conclusions are only tenuous at this point because of several limitations with the research conducted to date. First, most of the research has consisted largely of uncontrolled case studies. Therefore, it is difficult to draw conclusions about the general population of anxious people with an ASD on the basis of reported results from one or two people only. Second, none of the studies have included a control group or placebo condition. Therefore, there has been no way of knowing whether the medication reduces anxiety symptoms better than no treatment at all or taking a sugar pill. Third, in the studies noted, often objective or standardized assessment measures were not used to measure the treatment results. Rather, clinical observations were reported. Therefore, it is difficult to have an objective sense of any improvement in anxiety symptoms without objective measures being used. Fourth, the effects of medication only appear to last as long as the medication is being consumed with the chance of relapse occurring once the medication regime is ceased (Tsai, 1999).

Guidelines for Using Medication to Treat Anxiety Disorders

Medications are not the full or only solution for anxiety treatment.

It is important to note that medications are not a complete treatment for many anxiety disorders. That is, often medication alone will not totally resolve a person's anxiety difficulties. Rather, effective treatment involves many of the indirect treatment strategies discussed in Chapters 5 and 6 in this book as well as many of the cognitive behavioral strategies discussed next in Chapter 8. Perhaps the best way to consider medication is as a means for the anxious person to learn to assist herself. In other words, medication is typically best utilized when it is part of a holistic treatment program that involves changes and support within the person's environment as well as strategies to face and conquer her fears and develop more self-confidence.

Obtain an accurate diagnosis.

It is important to avoid the temptation to diagnose your own child but to ensure that her anxiety difficulties are assessed properly, as discussed in Chapter 1. Once a thorough assessment is complete, then an accurate diagnosis can be made regarding the specific type of anxiety disorder or problem a person has. In turn, better decisions can be made regarding treatment planning including what specific medications might be worth considering as a part of that treatment plan.

There are no magic pills or cures.

Medication will not remove all of a person's anxiety difficulties, take away all her symptoms, or remove the source or object of her fear. For example, medication cannot remove the dogs on your street if you have a child with autism who is fearful of dogs. Similarly, it might not make your child feel comfortable enough to suddenly approach and pat a dog. All professional interventions, whether individual therapy, group therapy, medication, behavioral techniques, or practice exercises, have the same focus: to build the person's own belief in herself;

that she is the best person to control her own fears and develop her own self-confidence. Unfortunately, sometimes the person with anxiety, her family, and the professionals who work with her might surrender themselves to anxiety, believing that the way to manage it is somehow beyond their own control. In believing this, then we are also reducing the individual's self-esteem, determination, and her willingness to trust herself. Rather, this person might develop an unhealthy dependence on medications, physicians, other professionals, friends, and family.

Medication is not a "weak" or toxic solution.

Alternatively, some families—certainly many parents I work with—tell me that medication is for "weak" people and they do not want their son or daughter to end up reliant upon it. Or, that the side effects of medication are so detrimental that their child will experience a "toxin" in her system. While such fears are understandable, they are not always realistic. Medications are not designed to poison the individuals taking them; rather they are carefully manufactured to assist those individuals. Moreover, those that prescribe them have years and years of training and experience in finding and monitoring appropriate medication regimes. Not all people taking medication experience side effects. In addition, sometimes the benefits of medication outweigh the possible side effects, especially in the instance of severe or debilitating anxiety (the kind that can lead to depression). What we know from science and research is that medications might be effective and appropriate depending on the particular problem that a person experiences. That is, they are best not ruled out completely until a clear understanding of the person's type of anxiety difficulties is established.

Do not self-medicate.

As I stated at the outset of this chapter, I am not a physician; therefore, I do not have the expertise to suggest dosages and types of medications to my clients. If you consider medication as an option in a treatment plan, I would certainly recommend that you seek the expertise of the appropriate medical professional, namely, your general practitioner, pediatrician, or psychiatrist. It is very important that, if choosing to include medication in a treatment plan, it is adopted under supervision of a medical professional and according to her advice. Key points include:

- giving the medication a fair trial to allow enough time to adequately determine the benefit of any medication;

- working with your medical professional, especially in the early weeks of a medication trial, to adjust the dose and to relieve any worries you might have about taking the medication; and
- following the prescription determined by the medical professional rather than raising or lowering dosages according to your own ideas, what other nonmedical professionals suggest or, worst of all, what you read about on the Internet!

Be prepared to experience side effects.

Most medications are associated with side effects. Side effects of anti-anxiety medications can include:

- Upset stomach
- Blurred vision
- Headache
- Confusion
- Grogginess
- Nightmares
- Dizziness or lightheadedness
- Nausea
- Nervousness
- Excitement
- Trouble sleeping
- Fatigue
- Cold hands
- Weakness

Some medications can worsen symptoms associated with asthma or diabetes if the individual suffers with either or both of these chronic conditions. In other instances, it can be hard to tell if the medication is working since some of the side effects mimic the very symptoms of anxiety. So if you opt to try medication as an intervention for anxiety, be guided by your physician in "sticking it out" so that, beyond the possible side effects, you can see if there are discernable benefits. Often, the side effects listed above are experienced in the early days or weeks of taking the medication rather than being long-lasting. Again, the experience of side effects and any need for advice or help in managing them highlights the need for anyone who is taking anti-anxiety medication to be in frequent contact with her physician rather than manage her medication dosages herself.

Discuss lowering doses with the medical professional as the person with ASD progresses with her treatment plan.

Typically, as a person progresses with direct treatment of her anxiety difficulties and becomes better able to face her fears and cope, then lessening her dosage of medication might be appropriate. For example, when a person begins "exposure tasks," as described next in Chapter 8, it is important that the person is able to truly experience the full extent of her anxiety in order to use her own skills to manage, rather than rely on, an altered experience of anxiety because of her medication. However, it is equally important for clinicians to communicate and work together when this occurs. For example, if a clinical psychologist begins exposure tasks at the same time as the person is taking anti-anxiety medication, then both the clinical psychologist and the physician need to communicate to determine what the best plan will be regarding lowering the patient's dosage.

Cease the use of medication gradually.

I often work with families who tell me that they simply stopped their child from taking her anti-anxiety medication without consulting the prescribing medical professional. In general, many of the anti-anxiety medications described in this chapter are best tapered off slowly to avoid any difficulties such as withdrawal symptoms. That is, it is important that you do not suddenly or abruptly discontinue a daily dose of a medication without first consulting the trained medical professional who has prescribed it.

In Summary

- Until recently, only two main forms of treatment were used to target anxiety difficulties in people with autism: psychoanalytic therapies and medication.
- Psychoanalytic therapies lack strong scientific evidence to support their use. Studies only used very small numbers of participants to explore the benefits of psychoanalysis.

- Psychoanalytic therapies also tended to be based on the now discounted notion that autism is somehow caused by poor bonding between a mother and her child.
- Other alternative therapies such as art and play therapy lack scientific evidence for their use in directly targeting the core difficulties of anxiety in people with an ASD.
- The use of complementary and alternative medicine for people with autism seems to have gathered support and momentum in the past few years and include:
  - Special diets
  - Extra vitamins or minerals
  - Food supplements
  - Herbal remedies
  - Massage and/or body-work therapies
- In general, scientists suggest that research regarding complementary and alternative medicine for people with autism needs to be interpreted with caution because of flaws in the methods used to carry out the research.
- Until the past few years, medication has been one of the most widely used treatments for anxiety in people with autism.
- The same medications that are prescribed for anxious individuals in the general population are also used to treat anxiety in people with autism. These medications include:
  - Benzodiazapines
  - Antidepressants
  - Beta-blockers
- These medications are used to treat a range of anxiety difficulties including:
  - Panic attacks
  - Obsessive Compulsive Disorder
  - Generalized Anxiety Disorder
  - Social Anxiety Disorder/Social Phobia
  - Simple Phobias/Specific Phobias
- At this stage, it is hard to determine how effective medication is in treating anxiety in people with autism. Anxiety seems to reduce only as long as medication continues to be taken.

- Some challenges exist within current research on medication such as the very small numbers of people investigated, the inability to make comparisons about whether medication is better than a placebo, and the tendency for results to be based on the researcher's clinical observations rather than a more objective assessment measure.
- If medication is used as a treatment for anxiety in a person with autism, then important guidelines need to be considered including:
    - that medication is used in conjunction with other forms of skill-based intervention;
    - that the person undergoes a thorough assessment of her exact anxiety difficulties before commencing any medication regime;
    - that emphasis is not placed on medication as a "cure" for anxiety difficulties; and
    - that families work closely with doctors and clinicians to ensure that medication regimes are followed as prescribed rather than determining themselves when to raise, lower, or cease dosages.

Direct Treatments for Anxiety:
Cognitive Behavior Therapy

Jeremy and the Fraser Family

Jeremy is seven years old, has autism and mild intellectual delay. "He seems constantly anxious about many activities," Jeremy's parents told me during our first consultation. "The main challenge at the moment seems to be about using the toilet. He refuses to sit on it and says that he is scared, but we can't seem to work out exactly what it is about using the toilet that makes him nervous. He has been wearing a Pull-Ups® diaper to school because he refuses to use the toilet there. However, the toilet is just one of many things that make him anxious. He worries about night-time, going to school, homework, places where there are a lot of other children and perhaps lots of noise, bees, and leaving the house to go on fieldtrips. There are probably other things we've forgotten; it's a long list." "What are your expectations in coming to see me?" I asked. "We've come here because we read about cognitive behavior therapy and we were told that it is one of your 'specialties.' We don't want to medicate our son so we thought we should try this." I asked what they had read. "We've read a book that suggests that CBT might be effective in teaching children how to reduce their own anxiety. We want Jeremy to learn skills to cope by himself. We're running out of ideas to try to manage him at home. We thought that if he could learn some ways to feel calmer and less worried, then it might be better than us always trying to tell him not to worry because that doesn't seem to work. But his classroom teacher told us not to bother with this therapy. She said that it won't work for Jeremy because he has autism and that you can't use it with children with autism. Then a friend told me that she had seen you and you do use it with children *with autism. We just want to know whether you think it might be worth trying with Jeremy. We're desperate!"*

It is always so interesting to discover what exactly has led a family to our clinic in Sydney, Annie's Centre. It fascinates me to learn about the reading and research that parents have completed before they've set foot in our centre. Moreover, I am curious about the people they have spoken to before coming to see me and the various opinions they have listened to from other parents or professionals regarding what they should or should not try in aiming to help their child. In a way, it reminds me of my own preparation ahead of the birth of my first child. I read books and sought information online. People were also very forthcoming with their opinions (founded and unfounded) regarding what I should eat, what doctors I should see, what exercise I should do, when I should take a break from work, what type of birth plan I should have, and many other pregnancy and birth-related issues. In general, it made me feel more nervous and anxious—not less; much like the Fraser family was feeling when they attended their first consultation.

My point is that just as the experience of a pregnancy is unique for each mother, so too is the experience of raising a child with autism unique for each family. Therefore, sometimes it is not helpful for other parents or professionals to make assertions regarding what treatment approach should be followed unless their assertions are based on some kind of solid, scientific evidence. When I tried to determine the best plans to make ahead of the birth of my first child, I wrote lists of questions and took them to the person considered the scientific expert for pregnancy and birth, my obstetrician. Together we discussed the evidence for and against options such as special diets, exercise regimes, birth plans, and related topics. After these discussions and listening to the scientific evidence, I felt more comfortable making my own decisions.

As we've seen in Chapter 7, when it comes to the scientific research for anxiety treatment for people with autism, it is limited at best. We still do not know very much about how well treatments such as psychotherapy, special diets, and medication work. We need to see more research in these areas as they are still in their infancy.

Another treatment we are still learning more about (as were the Frasers) is cognitive behavior therapy (CBT). CBT has existed for decades and has been scientifically shown to be very effective in treating anxiety in typically developing people. However, we've only recently begun to see some evidence that CBT might also be effective in treating anxiety in people with an ASD. This chapter outlines the key components of CBT, the related CBT techniques that you can use with your child, student, or client, and examples of exactly how to implement these CBT techniques in therapy, school, and the home.

As the Fraser family noted, CBT is one of my "special interests." Indeed, colleagues at the Centre for Emotional Health at Macquarie University, Sydney, and I developed a manualized treatment program for anxious individuals with autism. If you are a professional who is interested in using CBT with your anxious ASD clients, then I strongly recommend you look at the full treatment program, *Cool Kids® Child Anxiety Program: Autism Spectrum Disorders Adaptation* (Chalfant, Lyneham, Rapee & Carroll, 2011). Many of the concepts and strategies discussed in the current chapter are presented in further detail in that program. Some concepts and images have been reproduced in this chapter with permission from the authors. The *Cool Kids® Child Anxiety Program: Autism Spectrum Disorders Adaptation* is available from our clinic, Annie's Centre and from the Centre for Emotional Health at Macquarie University in Sydney (details for both centers are provided in the Appendices).

What is Cognitive Behavior Therapy?

Cognitive behavior therapy (CBT) is a psychological approach that aims to solve problems involving dysfunctional emotions, behaviors, and cognitions. It is goal-focused and systematic in its approach. CBT has been used in various forms since the 1960's to help treat a variety of problems including mood, anxiety, personality, eating, substance abuse, and psychotic disorders. Treatment using CBT is often "packaged" into step-by-step manuals or guides with sets of instructions/guidelines for treatment of specific psychological disorders. The guidelines instruct the clinician or therapist regarding exactly what strategies and skills to cover and how within each session of his treatment programs. CBT is used in individual therapy as well as in group settings. During theses sessions the client/patient is taught skills to ultimately learn to help himself.

CBT is based on the premise that the characteristics of psychological problems like anxiety symptoms are related to the interaction of thoughts, behaviors, and emotions. Therefore, in CBT, the therapist and patient/client work on identifying and directly changing thoughts and behaviors that may be maintaining the symptoms. The therapist often assigns homework for the patient to complete outside of his therapy sessions to ensure that the person practices the skills he is learning. Patients/clients typically attend sessions regularly for up to several months in order to develop skills to combat their difficulties. Then, they begin to phase out therapy with a view to independently implementing the skills learned. You might recall that Jeremy learning to "help himself" is exactly what the Fraser family was seeking for their son so that he could become more independent of them in managing his own anxiety.

In relation to anxiety disorders, CBT seeks to address the worried thinking (cognitions) and the avoidance (behavior) that are characteristic of anxiety. These characteristics were outlined in detail in Chapter 1.

Basic Components of Cognitive Behavior Therapy in Treating Anxiety Disorders

Treatments from a cognitive behavioral perspective assume that anxiety is comprised of a biological, behavioral, and psychological component (e.g., Albano & Kendall, 2002). Therefore, CBT for anxiety disorders typically involves four key components that address the biological, behavioral, and psychological difficulties associated with anxiety. The four treatment components are:

1. *Education:* Information about anxiety and the difference between normal and abnormal, or helpful and unhelpful, anxiety.

2. *Relaxation skills:* Teaching relaxation skills to target the autonomic arousal and associated physiological responses of unhelpful anxiety, e.g., the symptoms of hyperventilation, racing heart rate, and muscle tension.

3. *Cognitive restructuring:* Exercises that focus on identifying threat-focused, maladaptive thoughts. People are taught how to replace or restructure these thoughts by adopting a helpful or "brave" thinking style.

4. *Graded exposure:* Developing a hierarchy of feared activities, situations, or objects that might be avoided. Conducting exercises to gradually face fears on the hierarchy

while using the relaxation and cognitive restructuring skills already acquired.

Scientific Support for CBT

Is There Any Scientific Support for CBT as a Direct Treatment for Anxiety Disorders?

Researchers and clinicians have begun to consider the use of CBT to treat anxious people with autism because of the very large body of scientific evidence that already supports using CBT to treat anxiety in typically developing individuals, across all ages. Therefore, it is important to have a closer look at the evidence for CBT with typically developing people to better understand why clinicians like myself are so keen on trying to apply it to people with an ASD. Most of the reviewed research below focuses on the use of CBT to treat anxiety in children and adolescents as parents and professionals reading this book might be most concerned about these age groups.

Studies Looking at the Use of CBT vs. a Wait-list Control Group

Some of the earliest evidence for the efficacy of CBT in treating anxiety disorders in typically developing children comes from a study by Kendall (1994) using a manualized CBT intervention he developed with colleagues called the "Coping Cat" program. Kendall (1994) found that the majority of the forty-seven anxious children assigned to the treatment condition no longer met criteria for an anxiety disorder after CBT treatment. Specifically, the majority (64 percent) of the treatment group no longer had an anxiety disorder compared to only one child in the untreated group on the waiting list for the program. These findings were based on both clinical observations and a range of symptom checklists given to the children pre- and post-treatment (Kendall, 1994). Follow up assessment indicated that the treatment gains had been maintained after one year (Kendall, 1994). Moreover, a recent long-term follow up study revealed that the treatment gains continued to be maintained seven years after the initial treatment (Kendall, Safford, Flannery-Schroeder & Webb, 2004). That is, the CBT program seemed to be of long-term benefit to the children who participated.

A second evaluation of the "Coping Cat" program was again conducted by Kendall et al. in 1997. They assigned sixty children (aged nine to thirteen years) to a treatment group and thirty-four to a waiting-list. As in their first study, they found that post-treatment, 54 percent of the treated group was free of an anxiety disorder diagnosis compared with only 6 percent of those on the waiting list (Kendall et al., 1997). Significant improvements were again found in symptom severity for those in the treatment group based on both self- and parent-report measures (Kendall et al., 1997). As with the original study, one year follow-up data revealed the maintenance of treatment gains (Kendall et al., 1997).

Barrett, Dadds & Rapee (1996) adapted Kendall's treatment program for an Australian population and incorporated a family treatment component. As a result, parents attended a joint parent-child session each week to develop collaborative strategies to help manage their child's anxiety in the household. Similar to Kendall's findings, significant post-treatment reductions in anxiety occurred for all those in the CBT groups, with greater reductions occurring for those who attended the combined CBT-Family treatment condition (Barrett et al., 1996). The results were maintained at six and twelve month follow-up periods with 95.6 percent of the CBT-Family treatment group being diagnosis free twelve months after treatment completion (Barrett et al., 1996). In fact, a more recent longer-term follow-up indicated that 85.7 percent continued to remain diagnosis free six years after the CBT treatment (Barrett, Duffy, Dadds & Rapee, 2001).

Kendall's program was also adapted in order to be delivered to small groups of children (approximately three to six children per group) by Silverman et al. (1999). When evaluating the group model of CBT delivery, Silverman et al. (1999) found significant improvements for children in the treatment groups at post-treatment as well as at three, six, and twelve month follow-ups. Seventy-six percent of the children who completed the group-based CBT program remained anxiety diagnosis free twelve months after program completion (Silverman et al., 1999).

From these studies it seems reasonable to conclude that for children and adolescents there is good scientific support for the use of CBT as a direct treatment for anxiety disorders.

CBT and Anxiety Prevention

Not only has CBT been shown to be effective in **treating** anxiety symptoms in children, but also, more recently, CBT has been found to be effective in **preventing** the development of anxiety symptoms in children (see Barrett & Turner, 2004 for a review). For example, Barrett and Turner (2001) developed a twelve-session CBT intervention called the "Friends for Children" program that could be incorporated into classroom curriculum as a means of preventing anxiety. They (2001) assessed the efficacy of the preventative intervention using a sample of 489 primary school-aged children. The intervention was found to reduce the report of anxiety symptoms (Barrett & Turner, 2001).

CBT as an "Efficacious" Treatment

The evidence supporting CBT for typically developing anxious people is so strong that CBT was deemed an "efficacious" treatment by the "Committee on Science and Practice" (Chambless & Hollon, 1998). The Committee on Science and Practice is an initiative of the Society of Clinical Psychology, a division of the American Psychological Association. It was developed to help educate consumers about the most evidence-based psychological interventions. This milestone in recognizing CBT as a good treatment option for anxious people was based on several criteria set out by the committee. Essentially, the committee deemed that the research on CBT is exemplary in five ways. First, research has included cases serious enough to warrant formal diagnosis of an anxiety disorder and has employed standardized assessment tools in determining these diagnoses. Second, randomized control trials have indicated significant benefits of CBT treatments compared with wait-list control conditions. Third, research has indicated that the anxiety reduction attained from CBT programs has been maintained over long, post-treatment follow-up periods. Fourth, the superiority of CBT as a treatment for anxiety in children has been demonstrated by independent research groups in at least two different countries: the USA (Kendall et al., 1997) and Australia (Barrett et al., 1996). Fifth, most of the CBT programs evaluated have employed treatment manuals. Therefore, they have helped ensure better consistency in how the treatment has been delivered. It is interesting to note the contrast between the quality of CBT research regarding typically developing anxious people and that of some of the studies exploring psychotherapy, alternative medicine, and medication for people with an ASD outlined in Chapter 7.

Is There Any Scientific Support for Using CBT as a Direct Treatment for Anxious People Who Have Autism?

Studies Looking at the Use of CBT vs. a Wait-list Control Group

Although cognitive behavior therapy (CBT) has widely demonstrated efficacy among typically developing anxious children and adolescents (Albano & Kendall, 2002; Mendlowitz, Manassis, Bradley, Scapillato, Miezitis & Shaw, 1999; Shortt, Barrett & Fox, 2001), until the past five years, there has been little published literature regarding the use of CBT models to directly target anxiety in children or adolescents with autism. Some single case studies documented the use of modified CBT to address the behavioral difficulties associated with autism (e.g., Beebe & Risi, 2003). However, until recently, there was little published literature on clinical trials of CBT to specifically address anxiety in people with an ASD. CBT-like strategies were used indirectly by focusing on the parents. CBT was used to teach the parents how to manage their own stress and, in turn, cope more effectively with their children's anxious behaviors (Verheij & Van Loon, 1993). It was also used to teach the parents anxiety-reducing skills so that they could re-teach the skills to their children, thereby becoming their children's own therapist (Verheij & Van Loon, 1993). While there are documented benefits for including parents in anxiety interventions for children (Mendlowitz et al., 1999; Shortt et al., 2001), failure to include the children as direct participants in the intervention might result in less effective therapy. It might not only hinder the children's ability to become independently aware of their anxiety difficulties, but also their ability to independently manage them.

Some research evaluating the direct application of CBT in treating anxiety in people with autism has been conducted with promising results (White et al., 2009). Remission of anxiety disorders using CBT now appears to be an achievable goal at least among children with autism who are high-functioning. Several key studies have pioneered the use of CBT as a direct treatment for children with anxiety and autism. As an aside, I note proudly that two of these pioneering studies were conducted by Australian researchers!

First, Sofronoff, Attwood & Hinton (2005) evaluated the impact of a six-week CBT intervention for seventy-one school-aged children with Asperger's disorder. Children were randomly assigned to either a child intervention program, an intervention program for both children and their parents, or a waiting list. The intervention was delivered weekly in a group format. Coping strategies such as a "toolbox" of techniques that children could use to "fix" anxious feelings were taught during the weekly sessions. Focus was also placed on expanding emotional knowledge in the children by comparing emotions in different situations. The results indicated a reduction in parent-reported anxiety symptoms for the children at the six week follow-up after the intervention. Children who attended either intervention group also seemed better able to generate strategies for managing anxiety than those in the waiting list group.

Second, a study I conducted along with colleagues from Macquarie University and Autism Spectrum Australia (Aspect) (Chalfant, Rapee and Carroll, 2006) evaluated a family-based CBT treatment for anxiety in forty-seven children with comorbid anxiety disorders and high functioning autism and Asperger's disorder. Treatment involved twelve weekly group sessions. The children in the treatment group were compared with children who received no treatment that were on the waiting list for the program. Changes between pre- and post-treatment were examined using clinical interviews as well as child-, parent-, and teacher-report measures. Following treatment, 71.4 percent of the treated participants no longer fulfilled diagnostic criteria for an anxiety disorder. Comparisons between pre- and post-treatment indicated significant reductions in anxiety symptoms for the treated group as measured by all the self-report, parent-report, and teacher-report scales.

Most recently, studies from researchers in the United States have provided further support for the use of CBT in directly treating anxiety in children with autism. For example, Reaven et al. (2009) evaluated a CBT intervention with thirty-three children with high functioning autism and their parents. Results indicated significant reductions in the parents' report of anxiety symptoms after the delivery of the group treatment compared to the children who remained in the waiting-list control condition. Similarly, Wood et al. (2009) tested a modular (CBT) program with forty children with autism. A standard CBT program was augmented with extra treatment components designed to address the social and adaptive skill deficits of children with autism that might pose barriers to anxiety reduction. They found that 78.5 percent of the CBT group improved (i.e., presented with reduced anxiety) compared with only 8.7 percent of the wait-list group. Finally, White et al. (2010)

have begun to look at the use of a manual-based cognitive-behavioral treatment program to target anxiety symptoms as well as social skill deficits in adolescents with ASD, referred to as "Multimodal Anxiety and Social Skills Intervention" (MASSI). They have shown initial evidence for treatment feasibility with four adolescents. Consequently, a more in-depth trial of the intervention is currently underway with a larger group of adolescents.

CBT and Single Case Reports

CBT has also been explored in research using single case reports for children and adolescents with autism and a comorbid anxiety difficulty such as Obsessive Compulsive Disorder (OCD) and Social Anxiety Disorder. Again, there seems to be preliminary evidence to support the application of CBT to treat anxiety difficulties in people with autism. For example, Reaven and Hepburn (2003) successfully used CBT to treat OCD in a seven-year-old girl with Asperger's disorder. Similarly, Lehmkuhl et al. (2008) reported on the successful treatment of a twelve-year-old boy with autism who presented with OCD. Finally, Sze and Wood (2007) demonstrated successful outcomes when CBT was used to treat an eleven-year-old girl with anxiety and high functioning autism.

In conclusion, it seems fair to suggest that while the research for using CBT with people with an ASD is still emerging, there have been some good studies to date that suggest that it can be applied to people with an ASD, particularly to those people who are high functioning.

CBT Tools and Techniques

As described above, the four key components of most CBT programs for anxiety are:

- Education about emotions and anxiety
- Relaxation skills training
- Cognitive restructuring
- Graded exposure tasks

These components involve a range of tools and techniques to help the anxious person learn skills to overcome the core features of his anxiety: physical anxiety, anxious thinking, and avoidant behavior. Trained and experienced clinicians work with clients/patients to teach them skills in each of the above four components of therapy. There are now some examples of CBT-based intervention programs that have been produced into manuals with step-by-step instructions for how clinicians can implement CBT with their clients with an ASD. As mentioned above, you can find a good example of a CBT program and complete manual for treating anxiety in individuals with autism in the new *Cool Kids® Child Anxiety Program: Autism Spectrum Disorders Adaptation.*

Outlined below are a wide range of cognitive behavioral strategies to use with anxious people with autism. You might like to adapt some of these strategies for use with your children, students, or clients. As a rule of thumb, it is imperative that parents are involved in all strategies to help reduce anxiety in their children so that they can work alongside their children and support them in implementing any cognitive behavioral skills learned. The strategies and tools covered in this chapter are designed to be as practical as possible. Parents, teachers, and other professionals can use them to immediately start managing anxiety in their children, students, or clients without further assistance required from a mental health professional (e.g., psychologist). However, it is important to involve the expertise and skills of a trained professional if you believe that the person's anxiety difficulties are more severe. (How to judge the extent of someone's anxiety difficulties was outlined in Chapter 1.)

Education about Emotions and Anxiety

Before skills can be taught and used to combat symptoms of anxiety or worry, the person needs to learn how to recognize his own emotions. "If I can't recognize when I am feeling worried or anxious, then how am I going to know when to implement a strategy to reduce my anxiety? How can I tell the difference between worry and other emotions, for example, sadness or frustration?" Many CBT programs begin with emotion education. Usually, a wide range of emotions and related experiences are taught before honing in on specific feelings of fear or anxiety. There are many strategies that you can adopt to help a child, student, or patient become better aware of his emotions.

Education about Emotions
"Mind Reading" Games. Take turns displaying emotions using facial expression and whole body movements, for example, displaying an angry face at the same time as stomping a foot and folding arms

suddenly across the body. Ask your partner to try to guess the feeling or emotion that you expressed. Then swap roles and ask him to be the one to display an emotion using his facial expression and whole body movements, while you try to guess what emotion he is trying to convey. You can give him on-the-spot feedback and coaching to ensure that he learns how to make the right expression for each emotion. A point scoring system can be used with each person getting a point every time he correctly guesses an emotion. As individuals with ASD can have difficulty recognizing expressions, you can limit the activity to two or three very distinct emotions (e.g., happy/excited, sad, afraid) to begin with and then build up over time to a wider range including more subtle emotions (e.g., bored, disgusted, amused, surprised, curious, confused). The game can also be made more challenging by guessing emotions when displayed with facial expression and upper body gestures only, for example showing a surprised face while bringing hands up to either side of one's face to emphasize the feeling of surprise. Eventually, you can move on to guessing emotions that are displayed with facial expression alone.

Role Playing. Ask the client to think of an emotion or ask him to close his eyes and pick an emotion word (e.g., happy, sad) from a bag or hat. Then, ask the person to act out a sequence of events that might relate to that emotion. For example, if he were to pick the emotion "happiness," then he might be able to act out a situation when he felt happy, e.g., receiving a gift, visiting a friend, eating something he enjoys, or listening to his favorite song.

Emotion Worksheets or Flash Cards. Some people who are more significantly affected by autism might benefit from worksheets that incorporate their favorite cartoon characters, celebrities, friends, or family members showing various emotions, or flash cards on which a range of emotions are displayed using pictures or photos of them. Essentially, the activity here is learning via repetition which faces represent which emotions. You can shuffle the flash cards and then display them one at a time for the person to state the correct emotion for the card. Alternatively, you can prepare a worksheet by assembling photos or cut-out pictures of characters, celebrities, friends, or family and assembling them into rows on the paper so that each row represents a variety of emotions. Then, going along the rows, you can discuss and write down which emotion corresponds with which picture on the worksheet. For children who are verbal, you can then ask them to think of and tell you about a time when they have felt that emotion.

Video Modeling. Another technique that might be helpful for children who need more support is to use video footage of yourself. Act out and then play back various emotional responses with facial expression alone or with facial expression and other physical gestures. Show video snippets repeatedly to help teach the person with anxiety which emotions belong with each observed expression on the video. Using this as a tool, you can then train the person to demonstrate emotional responses himself by copying your behavior from the footage. Then try videotaping his expressions! A good resource is *Seeing is Believing: Video Self-Modeling for People with Autism and Other Developmental Disabilities* (Woodbine House, 2009).

Computer Programs. Some computer software has now been developed to assist people with an ASD in recognizing and understanding emotions. For example, *Mind Reading: An Interactive Guide to Emotions* (Jessica Kingsley Publishers, 2003) is a software program that explores the full spectrum of emotions. By using video footage, audio recordings, pictures, quizzes, and interactive games, a person can study emotions as well as learn which types of facial expression and tone of voice accompany various emotional experiences. Developed by Professor Simon Baron-Cohen, the program covers over 400 emotions that can be seen and heard performed by six different people. Games are included to help the person consolidate his learning.

> ### Tips:
> 1. Anxiety, fear, or worry are emotions that you would need to include in all of the games or tasks listed here as well as other common emotions such as anger, sadness, and excitement.
> 2. I would use the term "worry" with a client as it seems to be a simpler concept to understand than anxiety.
> 3. It is essential that the person learns to automatically recognize or describe the various emotions he experiences before you start working on other strategies to reduce worry or anxiety.
> 4. It is always important to reward the person using praise, affection, or more concrete rewards (e.g., stickers or time on the computer) whenever he makes an *effort* to label or identify emotions in himself or others.

Education about Anxiety

After you have established that your child, student, or client has expanded his understanding of emotions and can recognize emotional responses within himself, the next step is to provide more detailed information about the specific emotions of worry, fear, or anxiety. Below are some strategies for detailed education about worry or anxiety and their effects. Some descriptions are provided from the *Cool Kids® Child Anxiety Program: Autism Spectrum Disorders Adaptation*; however, they are just descriptions and suggestions to give you some idea of how to create your own activities and tasks. Using the following strategies, you can make up your own version of these sorts of activities that are more individualized for your own child, student, or client:

Puppets or Cartoon Characters. Using puppets or cartoon characters is a good way to engage people in the task of identifying worry or anxiety. For example, in the *Cool Kids® Child Anxiety Program: Autism Spectrum Disorders Adaptation* (Chalfant, Lyneham, Rapee & Carroll, 2011) we use two characters, an anxious alligator named "Austin" and a confident crocodile named "Calvin" to teach participants the difference between feeling worried and feeling brave or confident. The puppets discuss (via the clinician) their different experiences of these feelings. The participants are then asked to try to identify any similarities between themselves and the characters. For older or higher functioning students, puppets might not be necessary. Cartoons that are drawn up into a sequence of events depicting feelings of worry vs. bravery might be enough. However, I have observed that even some older elementary school children find the use of puppets fun and engaging.

Why use animal or cartoon characters? Over years of clinical practice, I have noticed that children with autism seem to have a strong affinity for animals or their favorite cartoon characters. Indeed, I frequently observe instances where clients tend to relate better to animals and cartoon characters than they might toward their same age peers. They seem better able to demonstrate sympathy for an animal or cartoon character. This allows the person to learn more effectively which of the two emotions (worry or bravery) is more helpful.

Anxiety Information Worksheets. The use of two characters—one anxious, the other brave—can also be incorporated into educational worksheets about worry vs. confidence as we have done in the *Cool Kids® Child Anxiety Program: Autism Spectrum Disorders Adaptation*. The worksheets show pictorially all of the situations that one character fears, then provides opportunity for the child to circle any of those situations that he also fears or has in common with the anxious character. Based on my own clinical experience, anxious children find it easier to identify with another anxious character by circling what worries they have in common rather than by having to generate their own separate list of what worries them.

Worksheets might also be used to highlight how we can respond with different emotions even though the situation is the same. Again, in the *Cool Kids® Child Anxiety Program: Autism Spectrum Disorders Adaptation* (Chalfant, Lyneham, Rapee & Carroll, 2011), worksheets are used to show how "Austin the Anxious Alligator" responds with intense worry and fear, whereas "Calvin the Confident Crocodile" responds with bravery or confidence. The point of these types of tasks is to help raise the person's awareness about the limiting impact that anxiety can have. For example, by showing pictorially that a character became worried when he saw a dog, ran away, and missed out on having fun at the park, then we can discuss with the person how the character's worries stopped him from doing things that he might actually have liked to do, i.e., go to the park. Similarly, we can show pictorially how Calvin the Confident Crocodile's bravery allowed him to complete activities and attain some sense of satisfaction or accomplishment, e.g., being brave when he had difficult homework rather than giving up and getting in trouble at school for not finishing his work (Chalfant, Lyneham, Rapee & Carroll, 2011).

Worry Rating Scales. It is helpful to provide anxious people with tools to help them see that their experience of worry can occur to varying degrees. Worry scales, or thermometers, are one way to show this variation. (Figure 4 on the next page is an example of the worry scale/thermometer we use in the *Cool Kids® Child Anxiety Program: Autism Spectrum Disorders Adaptation*.) The different numbers on the thermometer represent different levels of worry or fear. Lower numbers represent lower levels of fear and elevated worry levels are illustrated by the higher numbers on the thermometer. If thermometers are too abstract for the child you're working with, then other simpler scales can be used such as traffic lights to show increasing worry as colors go from green (no or very low level of fear) to yellow (moderate level of fear) to red (high level of fear). Alternatively, a scale based on various facial expressions from cartoon drawings or from photos can be used. For example, you can use a scale of faces to show changes in levels of worry from feeling brave, to feeling confused, to feeling cautious, to feeling uncomfortable,

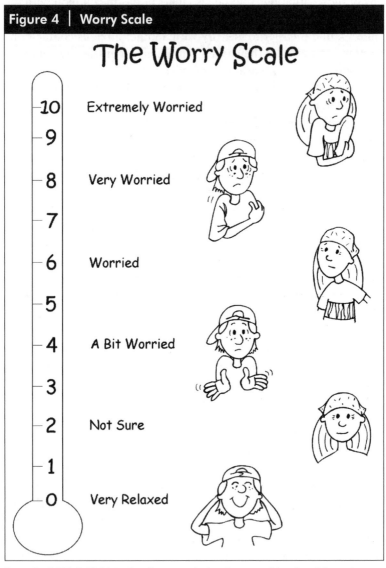

Figure 4 | Worry Scale

The Worry Scale

- 10 Extremely Worried
- 9
- 8 Very Worried
- 7
- 6 Worried
- 5
- 4 A Bit Worried
- 3
- 2 Not Sure
- 1
- 0 Very Relaxed

From *Cool Kids® Child Anxiety Program: Autism Spectrum Disorders Adaptation, Children's Workbook* by A. Chalfant, H. J. Lyneham, R. M. Rapee and L. Carroll, 2011, Macquarie University, Sydney: Centre for Emotional Health. Copyright 2011 by the Centre for Emotional Health. Reprinted with permission.

to feeling worried, to feeling panicked, to a full "meltdown" or panic attack. The use of worry scales/thermometers will be discussed again in more detail later in this chapter. These scales are designed to help people learn to be more aware and keep track of their own levels of anxiety. This is important because determining the degree of worry or anxiety they are experiencing helps them determine what kind of action/response to take, e.g., whether their anxiety level is low enough to be addressed by some simple relaxation skills or whether it is high enough to warrant an exposure hierarchy as outlined later in this chapter.

Body Awareness Activities. Before people can be taught relaxation skills to help combat their physiological experience of anxiety, they might need to improve their awareness of where in their body they experience anxiety. One engaging way to raise someone's awareness of his body reactions is to ask him to lie on a large piece of art paper and trace his silhouette. Then ask him to think about where in his body he notices a change when he feels worried or anxious and mark that part of his silhouette. For younger children, you can let them color in parts of a pre-prepared silhouette or drawing where they believe they feel anxious. You can also write some words for them to help describe their feelings. Alternatively, you can draw pictures to show the reactions, for example a cartoon picture of a heart running to show a "racing heart" or pictures of butterflies in the middle of the silhouette to depict the commonly reported experience of "butterflies in my tummy when I feel nervous." For older and higher functioning students, who might like to be more independent in completing this kind of task, you can use worksheets that already show a silhouette and simply ask them to mark the sheet themselves with colors, pictures, or words.

Monitoring Worry or Anxiety. To help ensure that an anxious person has regular practice at noticing his worries or anxiety, it is a good idea to use monitoring forms. Essentially, these can be like simplified diaries or tables to help identify when your child, student, or client felt worried and what he noticed within himself (i.e., in his body), as well as what happened in the end. For example, did he avoid the situation or object that he was worried about? Monitoring forms can be made as complicated or simple as required according to the client's level of functioning. For higher functioning individuals, you can use diaries with headings where they (or a parent if they do not wish to write) can fill in information covering: what day the worrying incident occurred, where it occurred, what happened, how worried they felt, any rating scale numbers or colors they might attribute to help show the extent of their feelings of anxiety, what they noticed in their bodies, and what happened in the end. An example of a monitoring form from the *Cool Kids® Child Anxiety Program: Autism Spectrum Disorders Adaptation* is provided in Figure 5. It is aimed at higher functioning individuals.

You can adapt this format to be even more pictorial and, therefore, more concrete for other children. For example, you could prepare a collection of pictures or photos that depict different objects or situations where the child tends to worry and his common reactions. That is, you could collect photos of the objects or situations, his facial expressions when worried or scared, his actions in terms of avoidance or challenging behavior, and any resultant consequences. Then you can lay these out all jumbled up across a table and ask the person to help you sort/order them appropriately to show you what happens first, then next, and so on.

For children with slightly higher support needs you could make the task even simpler by creating a visual sequence with cut-out pictures or photos and simply display them in the order they occur so that the person can see how one event of the sequence leads onto the next. This is similar to the way you might prepare a visual schedule or timetable but with the focus on experiencing worry. For example, if you are working with someone with high support needs who is afraid of storms, then you might create a visual sequence to show the following steps: hearing thunder, an expression of fear or worry, covering hands over ears, running away (e.g., to a bedroom).

For people with very high support needs (e.g., those with little or no spoken language), monitoring forms might not be appropriate. Rather, your own observations (e.g., from a functional behavior analysis) might be the best way to help you keep track of anxiety. Showing people at this level of functioning a visual sequence of their anxiety responses might cause them confusion and even serve to reinforce their anxiety. If you show a visual sequence, then they might incorrectly learn that this is how you *want* them to behave whenever they see the object of their anxiety.

Monitoring Worry within Classrooms or Small Groups.
Playing games in which you ask people to keep an eye out for "bossy worries" or spot worries within the classroom or a group can be a good

Figure 5 | Monitoring Form

Day	What was I worried about?	What did my body feel?	Parent Comment

From *Cool Kids® Child Anxiety Program: Autism Spectrum Disorders Adaptation, Children's Workbook*, by A. Chalfant, H. J. Lyneham, R. M. Rapee and L. Carroll, 2011, Macquarie University, Sydney: Centre for Emotional Health. Copyright 2011 by the Centre for Emotional Health. Reprinted with permission.

monitoring exercise for schools and therapy groups. You can ask the class or therapy group to watch for any "bossy worries" that the teacher/therapist displays or discusses. Naturally, the teacher/therapist needs to make some effort to frequently discuss and perhaps overdramatize worries or fears so that there is an opportunity for the class/group to pick up on them. For example, discussing and dramatizing fears of sudden noises, meeting new people, difficult work, crowds at the mall, animals, or insects can all provide opportunities for the group to observe and point out when a "bossy worry" was present and taking control. Using point systems to reward people who spot worries or identify fear in themselves or their peers might help motivate students to become better aware of worry and when it is occurring. Generally, if anxious people see these activities modeled on a whole class/group level, then they are more likely to feel comfortable applying the same process to themselves.

In general, all monitoring tasks help provide you with a means of seeing whether or not there are any patterns for the anxious person in terms of key situations or objects that seem to trigger anxiety. They also help you determine whether there are specific ways in which the person tends to respond. Information about these patterns is helpful in planning the use of relaxation skills and exposure tasks for the person.

Tips:

1. In general I have found that younger children and those who are lower functioning relate better to the phrases "feeling worried" or "feeling scared."
2. Terms such as "fear" or "anxiety" might be more appropriate for higher functioning individuals who are in the upper elementary to early high school years and for adolescents.

Relaxation Skills Training

Chapter 1 outlined detailed information about the physiological changes that occur when we experience fear or anxiety. Symptoms such as shortness of breath, sweaty palms, racing heart, and nausea were described. We know that rapid breathing often accompanies these symptoms. Therefore, many relaxation strategies that are used to help reduce anxiety target breathing, including:

Controlled Breathing Exercises

Essentially, controlled breathing is a skill that becomes easier with a lot of practice. If you are trying to teach this skill to a person with autism, I would strongly recommend that you encourage him to practice daily, several times each day (at least three times per day), and perhaps even prepare visual calendars and checklists to help him keep his practice up.

We all know how to breathe; however, controlled breathing is not as easy as it sounds. Typically, when I conduct controlled breathing sessions with clients with an ASD, I see that many people do not understand the concept of breathing in through the nose and out through the mouth. Most clients seem to breathe in and out using only one modality. Moreover, sometimes it is difficult for people with autism to count their own breathing cycles as they breathe and, therefore, to know when they are breathing too quickly or too slowly. That is why daily practice is so important. Controlled breathing does work well as a relaxation skill when someone is feeling anxious, but the person needs to learn to master the skill during regular practice sessions when he is not anxious for it to work effectively.

Controlled breathing (or you could call it "slow breathing," "calm breathing," or any other term that you think might be more appealing to your child or client) is easy to do anywhere and anytime because it focuses on breathing alone rather than any other physical activity like muscle relaxation exercises (described later). Therefore, it is easy to do controlled breathing without drawing attention to the anxious person. Often, I will tell young clients that it is a special kind of breathing, which they can do in secret (almost like magic breathing) so no one else will know when they are trying to calm down or get rid of worries in their body.

The key steps involved in controlled breathing are:

- making oneself comfortable;
- breathing slowly and evenly;
- breathing in through the nose and out through the mouth;
- breathing using six second breathing cycles (i.e., three slow counts to breathe in through the nose and three slow counts to breathe out through the mouth); and
- continuing using the breathing pattern until feeling calmer.

Again, it is very important that regular practice is emphasized. If you want your child, student, or client to implement breathing exercises as a relaxation skill, then you need to help him understand the value of regular practice. In my experience, children can be reluctant to practice breathing skills regularly (i.e., daily) because they are obviously not as much fun as spending time on the computer or being outside on the trampoline. However, as noted above, it is important to support practice with checklists, visual reminders, practice timetables, or reward systems so that the person is more motivated to try the technique.

I often encounter families at my clinic who tell me that they tried breathing exercises when their child was feeling anxious but that their child didn't really use them then and so they probably don't work. When I explore this issue further with the family, it usually becomes clear that they were only attempting to use the breathing techniques when their son or daughter was anxious rather than during scheduled practice times. Clearly, very little will change if you attempt to use a new skill only in the moments when you are feeling worried or anxious. Think of an alternative example: If you have to compete in a swimming race, you cannot expect that you will somehow be able to jump in the pool, swim a few laps, and place in the race if you have not been practicing swimming drills at regular practice sessions before the race occurs (e.g., doing laps with a kick board or practicing your stroke). It is the same with learning relaxation skills like controlled breathing. If the person with autism hasn't practiced the skill regularly when not feeling anxious, then he is going to be far less successful at trying to apply the skill when he actually does feel anxious. We've all experienced anxiety and how crippling it can be. It is hard, in the moment of feeling anxious, to think rationally enough to remember controlled breathing skills if they are not already automatic for us because of regular practice at other times.

Tips:
1. Controlled breathing is a skill that requires practice to learn how to do it well.
2. Make it a goal to practice controlled breathing daily, approximately three times per day.

Muscle Relaxation Skills

Often referred to as Progressive Muscle Relaxation (PMR), this relaxation strategy was first developed by Jacobson in 1938. PMR is a longer relaxation exercise that is easiest to complete either sitting or lying down. I usually suggest lying down to clients, but not on a bed where they might actually fall asleep. The PMR procedure teaches you to relax your muscles through a two-step process. First, you deliberately apply tension to certain muscle groups, and then you stop the tension and turn your attention to noticing how the muscles relax as the tension flows away. Essentially, PMR is about dividing the body up into various muscle groups and then, systematically, learning how to tense and release those muscle groups one at a time in order to gradually relax all parts of the body. Because the exercise takes longer to do and is less inconspicuous than controlled breathing, it is a good technique to use (on a daily basis) at home in the mornings before starting the day's routines and in the evening before the evening routines or before bed.

For younger and elementary school aged children, I often recommend that parents complete a PMR activity with their child before bed time. This creates a pleasant activity for the parent and child to do together. Completing a relaxing activity like PMR with a parent also helps motivate the child to learn the skill because he is likely to derive more enjoyment from doing it with his mom or dad than alone.

Key Steps in PMR

1. Find a quiet place with no distractions.
2. Remove your shoes.
3. Make yourself comfortable either sitting or lying down (on the floor).
4. Focus on controlled breathing (as described above).
5. Gently tense the muscles in the face and head as you breathe in and hold them in that tense position for a couple of seconds. Then slowly relax the muscles in the face and head as you breathe out.
6. Repeat the same steps above for the muscles of the neck and shoulders.
7. Continue the steps above in a slow and systematic way through the rest of the muscle groups in the body (see list of muscle groups below).
8. Once you have finished a full PMR exercise, count backwards slowly from ten to zero while remaining relaxed and engaging in controlled breathing for a few seconds before slowly getting up.

For higher functioning people with autism, the point of PMR is to help them focus on the change that occurs in their body as tension is let go so that they can learn subtle distinctions between muscular tension and muscular relaxation. It is important that you highlight this change for them as you move through each muscle group. For example, it is helpful to make statements like, "Hold your (insert muscle/ body part) in that position so it feels a little uncomfortable. Now, slowly relax your (insert muscle/ body part) and let the tension go. Feel the tension gradually leave your (insert muscle/ body part) bit by bit as you slowly relax it. Think about how your (insert muscle/body part) feels as the tension leaves it. It feels soft, floppy, relaxed. It feels so much nicer than feeling tense. Now focus on your breathing as your (insert muscle/ body part) stays relaxed."

You can choose to start with either top down sequences (i.e., face to feet) or bottom up (i.e., feet to face) sequences. At times, you might need to use a visual cue or gently tap the person on the particular body part if he has trouble identifying the area himself. To help you, the following is a list of muscle groups that you can use for PMR exercises with your child, student, or client:

- Right foot
- Right lower leg and foot
- Entire right leg
- Left foot
- Left lower leg and foot
- Entire left leg
- Right hand
- Right forearm and hand
- Entire right arm
- Left hand
- Left forearm and hand
- Entire left arm
- Abdomen
- Chest
- Neck and shoulders
- Face

One advantage of PMR is that it is a skill that can be used with flexibility. That is, the exercise can become as long or as short as required by including as many or as few different muscle groups from the list above as you think appropriate.

For more significantly affected children with autism, who might also have some intellectual delay, then body awareness can be more limited. Therefore, I might simplify the PMR exercise by grouping muscles together (e.g., do all the upper body at once by asking clients to give themselves a tight hug across their chest rather than trying to teach them to isolate their upper arms, chest, and shoulders). To begin with, you could also have them do the muscle work without the controlled breathing at the same time until they get the hang of the exercise. Alternatively, you can simply instruct them to take five slow, deep breaths at the start, in between each set of muscle tensing/relaxing movements, and again at the end so that the activity is a little more structured for them.

It is sometimes the case that clients with higher support needs engage in some type of repetitive behavior to self-sooth or relax (e.g., echolalia, stereotyped hand/finger mannerisms, or repetitive play with a preferred object). There is no reason why you can't incorporate some of these behaviors into a relaxation exercise. For example, allow them to repeat preferred phrases as they go through the PMR exercise or incorporate some of their repetitive movements into the muscle group movements of the PMR exercise before they relax them. However, in general, it is recommended that you try to teach them to substitute repetitive behaviors with more appropriate ways to relax. Again, using reward systems and positive reinforcement will help you teach them to increase their use of relaxation skills and reduce their use of repetitive behaviors.

There are many ways to develop picture sequences, checklists, and scripts as aides for completing PMR exercises. The *Cool Kids®* *Child Anxiety Program: Autism Spectrum Disorders Adaptation* contains a sample script for parents to use to help guide their child through the PMR exercise as well as worksheets with picture sequences to better explain the muscle groups used in the PMR exercises. You can, of course, make up your own picture sequences using your own visuals. You can also make up your own scripts by incorporating any special imagery that you know your child, student, or client might enjoy (e.g., asking him to imagine he is at a favorite park or beach). Some families like to use music to accompany PMR exercises. An Internet search will show you that there are hundreds of websites and resources out there for downloading or purchasing relaxation scripts and music to help in preparing your own relaxation activities. Whatever way you go about preparing relaxation resources is your choice; the main point is to include the key components of PMR as described above and then embellish the activity as you like to individualize it.

> ### Tips:
> 1. It is recommended that people practice PMR skills twice a day for approximately eight weeks before they can appreciate fully how to use it to relax independently.
> 2. For individuals who have high support needs, use picture sequences to help them see which body parts they are working on.
> 3. Consider incorporating a checklist system into the picture sequence so that someone can help check off each muscle group as the person completes the PMR step for that group.
> 4. For higher functioning teenagers, parents or professionals can record a brief script for the exercise to help the adolescents complete the exercise independently in their own time and in their own room.
> 5. For higher functioning individuals with autism, the point of PMR is to help them focus on the change that occurs in their bodies as tension is let go so that they can learn subtle distinctions between muscular tension and muscular relaxation. It is important that you highlight this change for them as you move through each muscle group.
> 6. If you are practicing at home, do not allow the person to complete the exercises lying down on a bed. Practicing in bed will increase the likelihood of the participant falling asleep and, consequently, he will derive little benefit from the sensation of being relaxed.

Cognitive Restructuring

Another CBT technique is called cognitive restructuring, which is essentially changing thoughts from negative or anxiety provoking to more positive or helpful. As discussed in Chapter 1, when someone is anxious or fearful, he is likely to experience worrying thoughts or "cognitions" about the object or activity that he fears. Typically, these thoughts involve overestimating the likelihood that the feared event will occur and catastrophizing how "bad" such an event might be if it is to occur. Consider a hypothetical example of my being fearful of speaking in front of other people. I might worry about being negatively evaluated or making a mistake. Therefore, if I had to deliver a presentation to an audience, then I might overestimate the likelihood of mistakes occurring and catastrophize that I am an incompetent speaker and that people in the audience feel that they wasted time in coming to listen to me present.

Usually, it is worried thinking that causes us to feel anxious—not the contents of the situation itself that we fear. To highlight this point, consider the examples in Table 9. There are various thoughts that I might have used in relation to giving a presentation. From Table 9 you can see that in the same situation of presenting to an audience, I might end up feeling quite different emotions and behaving differently, depending on how I think about the presentation. Therefore, if I want to overcome this anxiety, I need to aim to change my own thinking about the presentation rather than try to change or avoid the presentation itself.

Table 9	Possible Thoughts or "Cognitions" about Giving a Presentation		
Situation	**Thought**	**Emotion**	**Action**
Giving a presentation to a group of parents	I might make a mistake and appear as if I don't know my material well enough. They'll think I'm incompetent.	Anxious	Go over and over the presentation trying to perfect it. Or Take out the parts that I think lend themselves to my making a mistake.
Giving a presentation to a group of parents	I've prepared well for the presentation and so it's unlikely that I'll make a mistake. If I do make a mistake, then I can correct it. I'm sure the audience won't be bothered by it.	Calm or content	Deliver the presentation as planned.

Cognitive restructuring involves trying to shift the anxious person's thinking from what tends to be negative and unrealistic to calmer, more rational ways of thinking about a feared object or event. Given that cognitive restructuring involves working on people's thoughts, it might seem puzzling as to how this can be achieved with people with autism, who are considered to have core difficulties with abstract thinking and perspective-taking. However, as outlined in the research reviewed above, modified cognitive restructuring exercises have been shown to be very effective in the treatment of anxiety in people with high functioning autism and Asperger's disorder. Therefore, the examples of cognitive therapy skills and the exercises below pertain more to working with these groups than with those who are lower functioning or who also have some intellectual delay. Again, some of the strategies outlined below can be found in more detail in the *Cool Kids® Child Anxiety Program: Autism Spectrum Disorders Adaptation*.

Strategies to Help Teach the Difference between Worries and Helpful Thoughts

The following are ideas to jumpstart your efforts to teach anxious individuals with autism to distinguish between helpful thoughts and anxious ones. The *Cool Kids® Child Anxiety Program: Autism Spectrum Disorders Adaptation* also contains a range of examples of worksheets that you can use to help guide a person with high functioning autism or Asperger's disorder to do this as well.

- *Use pictures (e.g., colored pictures from favorite books, cartoons, or magazines, or computer generated) to help show the difference between helpful thinking vs. worries.* For example, use a picture of a person looking confident and calm for the helpful thoughts and a picture of a person looking nervous and fearful for the unhelpful thoughts. Place the pictures at the top of a whiteboard or large sheet of paper divided into two columns: one column for helpful thoughts, the other column for unhelpful thoughts. Then draw from a bag or hat a range of prepared (written or pictorial) worries and helpful thoughts, for example, "I'll never be any good at creative writing; it's too hard to think of what to write" (unhelpful thought), "The nine times multiplication tables are hard to remember, but I've learned the five times tables so I can do it again for the nines" (helpful). Ask the person to help sort the thoughts into either of the two categories: helpful or unhelpful. Give feedback to help correct any errors he makes if he allocates a thought into the wrong category.

- *If you work with groups of children, you could develop the same idea into a game by dividing the children into teams and allocating team points for each correct allocation they make.*

- *For older, higher functioning people, worksheets can also be developed to help show that someone can think about a situation in different ways.* For example, picture sequences can be used to show a feared object or situation, the person within the situation, and then two empty thought bubbles with visual cues to show which thought bubble is for the helpful thought and which thought bubble is for the unhelpful thought. The person would then be asked to generate ideas regarding what helpful or unhelpful thoughts might be written within each bubble.

- *Similarly, picture sequences can be used to depict an object or situation and a cartoon character's clear emotional reaction to that situation,* e.g., a look of fear in reaction to seeing a dog, a look of excitement in reaction to seeing another character, a look of anger in reaction to losing a game. Again, using empty thought bubbles, the person might then be asked to imagine and talk about what the character might have been thinking in each of the situations.

- *For younger kids or those in need of more support, you might fill in and read aloud the thought bubbles for them, then simply ask them to confirm for you which thought bubble represents a helpful thought and which represents an unhelpful thought.*

Tips:

Using your child's, student's, or client's favorite interests, TV shows, or book characters is helpful if you are developing booklets or worksheets to teach him the difference between worries and helpful thinking. For example, if a client is interested in the character "Harry Potter," then use images of Harry Potter in worksheets and related activities to engage him.

Using "Worry Stories" for Cognitive Restructuring

Once anxious people can better identify worries and helpful thoughts, they are likely to be ready to work on shifting or "restructuring" their worries into more helpful ways of considering an object or an event they fear. "Worry stories" were developed by myself and colleagues at the Centre for Emotional Health, Macquarie University, Sydney as a tool to help people with this process of "restructuring" (Chalfant, Lyneham, Rapee & Carroll, 2011). Again, there are several examples of worry stories in the *Cool Kids® Child Anxiety Program: Autism Spectrum Disorders Adaptation*.

In essence, worry stories are fictional stories about a character and an incident(s) where the character has experienced excessive worry and in turn coped badly (e.g., crying, avoiding, giving up) (Chalfant, Lyneham, Rapee & Carroll, 2011). The stories allow the person with an ASD to see how excessive worry can stop the character from coping and participating in activities he might otherwise be able to manage. The purpose of a worry story is to provide a means by which the person with an ASD can work on identifying unhelpful thoughts or worries and then come up with more helpful alternatives. They are a mechanism to teach cognitive challenging or restructuring.

Here are some tips for developing your own worry stories:

- Make them short, fun, and easy to read.
- Include pictures or illustrations.
- The storyline should describe a series of incidents where a character experiences worry because of how he interprets (or misinterprets) the situations he faces.
- Prepare the storyline using the preferred characters of the person with autism (e.g., preferred cartoon, film, or book characters).
- Base the storyline on any topic or event that you know causes anxiety for the person with autism. For example, if you know the person worries about swimming, then prepare a story about a swimming class. In the story, the character might avoid going in the water because of his worries and unhelpful thoughts about not being safe. At the end of the story he might miss out on having fun with the other students and feel frustrated and disappointed because his worries got the better of him.

- Try to include a range of unhelpful thoughts or worries that you know the person with autism tends to experience so that he can more easily relate to the story and engage in the identification of unhelpful thoughts or worries.
- Read the story aloud for the person. Ask him to listen very carefully like a "detective" so that he can tell you to "stop" when you read an unhelpful thought or worry.
- Each time you stop, have the person find and then underline in the story the unhelpful thought he has identified.
- Engage the person in a brief follow-up discussion regarding why the chosen thought is an example of a worried thought.
- Praise, encourage, and reward any efforts the person with autism makes to identify worried thoughts.
- Ask the person to generate examples of more helpful thoughts that the character in the story could have used to reduce his feelings or fear or anxiety.
- Prepare a range of worry stories to cover a range of situations so that the person has several opportunities to practice these skills.

Brave Thinking Lists or Booklets

For some people with autism, it might be too much to expect them to generate their own ideas of helpful thoughts to combat their worries. Most likely, this would be especially difficult for people who have language skills but are intellectually delayed. Therefore, you might need to provide them with cues, visual or otherwise, such as prepared lists or mini-booklets of common helpful thoughts from which they can choose rather than struggle to come up with their own ideas (see Table 10). Moreover, you can also develop miniature versions of the lists or booklets (e.g., pocket-sized, laminated cue cards or pocket books) for people to keep with them at all times so they have easy access to them as soon as they start to feel worried (Chalfant, Lyneham, Rapee & Carroll, 2011).

Brave thinking lists or booklets might be a suitable strategy not only for people with high functioning autism or Asperger's disorder but also for some people with autism who also have intellectual delay as outlined in the example below.

I consulted with a local elementary school regarding an anxious eight-year-old student with autism and mild intellectual delay. The student was particularly anxious regarding using the school toilets. Consequently, he would "hold it" all day until he was in the comfort of his own home to access a toilet. This type of avoidant behavior around toileting away from home is an issue that I come across frequently in my clinical work. A "brave thoughts" book was developed for the student to use whenever he was feeling worried (as identified by the student himself or as observed by his classroom teacher) about going into the school bathroom. Each page of the book contained a separate "brave" thought and, where possible, a picture to help convey the meaning of the brave thought. For example, the thought, "It's noisy in the school bathroom but the noise can't hurt me" was conveyed in words and pictures.

Other strategies such as relaxation skills (controlled breathing) and graded exposure tasks as described in the section below were also used. However, the point to emphasize here is that, even with a simplified format such as a list or booklet, it is possible to help a person with autism who has higher support needs learn some cognitive challenging strategies to combat worrying thoughts.

To help you develop your own booklets or lists for your own children, students, or clients, Table 10 provides some examples of both common worries and more helpful alternatives that I have noted from my own work with people with an ASD. No doubt, you can generate many others depending on the specific needs of the person you are supporting.

Role Playing

Role playing is another way to help people with autism better understand how to change their cognitions when anxious. Develop and act out scenarios wherein the person has been worried or scared and state out loud the unhelpful thoughts. Then ask the person to be like a movie director by telling you what brave or helpful thoughts to say aloud instead to help calm down and overcome the worries. Act out the related outcomes and actions of thinking more rationally about the feared situation.

If you work with groups of children, you can ask the children to form smaller groups. Have them collaborate to come up with new, helpful thoughts and then ask them to act these out within their groups to demonstrate how thinking the helpful thoughts allowed them to better overcome a worry.

Table 10 | Common Worries and Helpful Thoughts

Common Worries or Unhelpful Thoughts	Brave or Helpful Thoughts
I'm going to fail the test.	I need to try my best on the test.
I can't hand in my work unless Mom checks it over.	I am smart enough to give my work a try without Mom checking it for me all the time.
What if someone laughs at me during sharing time?	No one has laughed at me during sharing time before, but if they do, I can ignore them.
They'll think I'm weird if I try to speak to them.	They might be interested in talking to me. If not, it doesn't mean I've done something wrong.
I can't make any mistakes on my homework.	Mistakes help me learn. Everyone makes mistakes.
If I lose, then I must be dumb.	Everyone has a turn at winning and losing because everyone is good at different games.
The teacher might be angry with me if I don't finish all my work.	The teacher's job is to help me learn how to do my work—not get angry at me.
If I'm late, then I'll get into trouble.	If I'm late, I can take a late note. I probably won't get in trouble.
The dog will bite me.	Most dogs I've seen have been friendly and didn't bite me.
That food will taste terrible.	Even if the food tastes disgusting, it won't hurt me.
The noise sounds too scary and loud.	Loud noises don't sound very nice but they can't hurt me.
What if no one wants to play with me?	I can ask to join in. If that doesn't work, then I'll ask the teacher to help me find someone to play with.

Worry Diaries

Diaries might be suitable for older, higher functioning individuals, i.e., older children and adolescents with high functioning autism or Asperger's disorder. Essentially, worry diaries are sheets or booklets that you can prepare and give to your child, student, or client to help him keep track of worried thoughts and write down his brave or helpful thoughts to combat the worries. For example, you might ask a teenager to keep track of his worries with the following headings in a diary:

- What happened to make me worry?
- What worried thoughts did I notice? (You can provide a list of possibilities or leave the space empty for an older student to report his own.)
- How did that make me feel? (Provide a list of feelings from which he can circle the relevant emotion.)
- How did the worrying affect me physically? (You can provide a list of possibilities or leave the space empty for an older student to report his own.)
- What helpful thoughts could I have used to overcome the worried thought? (You can provide a list of possibilities or leave the space empty for an older student to report his own.)
- How does the helpful thought make me feel? (Provide another list or visual depictions of feelings for them to circle the relevant emotion.)

Graded Exposure Tasks

In Chapter 1, the impact of avoidant behavior on worry or anxiety was discussed. As described in that chapter, when a person avoids the object or event that worries him, he is teaching himself that he is safer away from that situation. In turn, he is preventing himself from learning that, if he did remain near the object or in the situation, then he could probably cope and be equally safe. Therefore, the fourth and very important element of most CBT programs for anxiety is tackling avoidant behavior. In CBT, this is done using a procedure called graded exposure.

Graded exposure involves systematically placing oneself in increasingly challenging situations that provoke anxiety. To achieve this, the person's fear is broken down into a series of smaller "steps" that, once achieved, allow the person to ultimately conquer the larger fear.

Completing exposure tasks can be challenging because it necessarily involves the person facing the object or event that he would otherwise like to avoid. Therefore, it typically involves increased levels of discomfort.

Why Expose Someone to Something He Fears, Knowing He'll Feel Uncomfortable?

Although exposure tasks involve an increase in discomfort to the person, we persist because we know it has three main benefits:

1. Exposure provides another means by which the person can see concrete or "live" evidence against an unhelpful thought or worry.

This is particularly beneficial for individuals with autism who benefit from concrete and visually clear examples to make learning experiences more salient. While the cognitive restructuring strategies described above provide skills to help shift irrational thinking, exposure tasks help provide concrete evidence that the brave thoughts might actually be true. For example, it would be hard to demonstrate that a worry like, "If I'm late to school, I will get detention" is incorrect if the child is never late to school (because he constantly avoids the experience of being late). Therefore, to help validate the braver thought, "I probably won't get a detention for being late to school," the person needs to have first-hand experience of what actually does occur when he is late, i.e., he needs to arrive late to school.

2. Exposure involves desensitization to feelings of anxiety.

"Desensitizing" or "habituating," when referring to anxiety, essentially means that the person "gets used to" or becomes gradually accustomed to the object or event he fears. Specifically, at a physical level, after repeated exposure to a feared situation, the body's reaction to that situation becomes calmer. For example, if you are startled when you see a barking dog, then, as discussed in Chapter 1, your body might experience anxiety symptoms such as racing heart, rapid breathing, and tensed muscles. However, if you were to come across the same barking dog every day, then the experience would become more familiar, and your body would stop reacting with the same degree of fear. Moreover, with less physical symptoms present, your mind would also be less likely to interpret the situation as worthy of anxiety. That is, your level of anxiety reduces. The anxiety levels also start to drop away faster. Therefore, as the person becomes more and more used to the object or event he fears, he seems to make bigger and faster gains.

3. Exposure builds confidence regarding the feared object or event.

The more the person has the opportunity to face his fears and "survive," the more his confidence will increase. Moreover, the more confident he feels, the more likely he is to be motivated to tackle the next step of exposure to other feared objects or situations. For example, I am currently working with a seven-year-old boy, named Evan, who has a diagnosis of autism and mild intellectual delay. He also suffers with Generalized Anxiety Disorder. He has a range of worries related to eating various fruits and vegetables, dressing himself, talking to other people, making mistakes or having errors marked as incorrect by a teacher, and water (e.g., swimming pools and the beach). The worst of these is his fear of water. Specifically, he fears going underwater and drowning. Prior to starting CBT and exposure tasks, Evan would not even discuss the idea of ever being able to swim in a pool someday. Evan and I determined that the easiest area for him to begin to face his fears was in relation to his fear of eating certain fruits. We then moved onto the issue of socializing and talking to strangers. Now, since Evan has begun to engage in the social exposure tasks successfully, he has developed more self-confidence in his ability to face his fears. Consequently, several weeks ago in a session with me, he asked, "Before I retire from working with you, will you be helping me to boss away my worries about swimming? What will the steps be on that stepladder?" Apart from the amusing choice of words regarding his future "retirement," what struck me was that he seemed interested in discussing what steps might be involved in tackling his worst fear. It is highly unlikely that Evan would have even considered listing out steps toward swimming if he had not already had some success with exposure to other worrying objects or events.

Steps in Setting Up an Exposure Program

To establish an exposure program, you need to develop a hierarchy of feared situations that the person will tackle one at a time. The exposure hierarchy is critical to ensure that there is gradual exposure to feared objects or situations rather than the person being overwhelmed by having to face his most feared situation first. The four steps in creating a hierarchy or "stepladder" of situations are outlined below:

1. Identify a Range of Feared Objects and/or Situations.

To help you determine the range of the person's worries or fears, you can develop a "worries list" that is broken up into sections according to which worries make the person feel **a little** worried or scared, which worries make the person **very** worried or scared, and which worries make the person **extremely** worried or scared. You might be able to develop the list from what you know of the person or you might ask the person to help you prepare the list, depending on his abilities. Where possible, it is very important to include the child and his parents in the preparation of the list so that the child is more likely to take ownership of any of the stepladders that are developed on the basis of the list. Table 11 is an example of a worries list from an anxious eight-year-old boy named Nathan who has high functioning autism. Naturally, your own children, students, or clients will have their own range of fears or worries. However, some of the issues in the worry list below do seem to be relatively common among individuals with autism.

From the worry list in Table 11 on the next page you can see that the ratings (out of 10) are included to help gauge how worried each situation makes the client feel beyond the qualitative descriptions in the left hand column. It is recommended that you do this in order to assist in developing a better range of anxiety provoking situations. Using the rating system above, a 0 (zero) rating would mean no worry at all and a rating of 10 would be the most worried. Of course, you can adjust the above list to make the information on it more pictorial for clients who benefit from visual cues. For example, collect pictures of the situations feared and then use a picture of a worry thermometer to help determine the relevant level of anxiety.

2. Determine Which Key Issues or Areas Your Stepladders Will Cover.

Once you have prepared the worries list, you can then categorize the worries and determine what kind of stepladders to create for the person. For example, from Nathan's list, I saw some common themes, so I grouped some of the items on the list into separate stepladders that cover broader topics. For example, Nathan identified feeling worried about eating meat, fruit, and vegetables. Therefore, I developed a stepladder that addresses the topic of trying new foods. Similarly, Nathan indicated feeling worried about talking to other children in class, playing with them, and going to birthday parties. I allocated

Table 11	Nathan's Worries List	
Level of worry I feel	**Situation**	**Rating (out of 10)**
Extremely worried	Birds	10
	Performing at assembly	9
	Going to a birthday party	9
Very worried	Eating vegetables	8
	Playing with other students during recess or lunch	7
	Eating fruit	6
	Presenting news to my class	6
A little worried	Eating meat	5
	Talking to children in my class	4
	Reading out loud in class	4

these fears to a single stepladder that addresses the broader topic of "socializing" or "making friends." Nathan also reported feeling worried about reading out loud in class, sharing news at circle time, and performing at assemblies. These worries could be put into a stepladder to address the issue of "performing in front of other people." Finally, since Nathan has reported feeling "extremely worried" about birds, I would develop a single stepladder to address this area, separately.

3. Develop the Steps That Go on Each "Rung" of the Stepladder.

The steps on the ladder must be ordered from the least scary (least distressing to tackle) as the first step to the most scary (most distressing to tackle) as the last step. Indeed, it is very important that you start with a first "step" that the person is relatively comfortable in completing so that he is always set up to succeed rather than be overwhelmed when he first begins exposure tasks. If a first step is too difficult for the person to achieve, then he might become so uncomfortable or distressed that he avoids the exposure task. It would be very difficult to build up to other exposure tasks after that experience. More than likely, the person would also feel that he had failed in some way and would lose self-confidence. A good example of the need to start with small and easy-to-manage steps comes again from Jeremy's mother, referred to at the start of this chapter.

If you recall, Jeremy has a long history of anxiety regarding toileting. He has difficulties in terms of body awareness and knowing when he needs to use the toilet. He is particularly anxious regarding using a toilet anywhere except in his home. At school, he "holds it" all day. His teachers and parents have been trying to address his anxiety regarding toileting at school.

After the family came to see me, we began a CBT program to address Jeremy's fear of toileting. Using an exposure hierarchy, we have been able to reach a level with Jeremy where he will enter the school bathroom on a regular basis with his peers at appropriate times in the daily routine. Therefore, we are now approaching the point of moving on to the next step on the hierarchy—using the toilet itself at school. Because of his difficulty with body awareness and tendency to have some toileting accidents, he wears Pull-Up diapers to school rather than regular underwear.

The school teacher called me last week to ask me whether it would be all right to make a contract with Jeremy as a part of his stepladder that the first step would be to attend school for a full day wearing normal underwear and not a Pull-Up. In my mind and Jeremy's mother's mind, this was an example of too big a first step on Jeremy's stepladder toward using the toilet at school. The best summary of this came from Jeremy's mother, who said, "If he was contracted to do this by his classroom teacher, then it would send him into such a state of panic that he would hardly be able to function at school during classes and he would begin to hate going to school altogether." In the end, we determined with the classroom teacher that smaller "no Pull-Ups" time segments during the day (e.g., thirty minutes) might be a more realistic starting point for Jeremy who was currently petrified of the idea of not having Pull-Ups available at school.

Jeremy's example highlights the need to spend adequate time and put careful planning into the stepladder process. It is important that the steps are small and gradual and that the starting point is achievable for the child to gain instant success with the process. Jeremy's example also highlights the need to work closely with school professionals when exposure steps need to be carried out at school. Sometimes extra "background" work has to be done at school to set up the steps, e.g., meeting with the classroom teacher and preparing (sometimes even involving) peers. From Table 12, you can see that some of the steps in a stepladder addressing a fear of public speaking incorporate the classroom teacher and responses from the children in the class.

To assist you in the process of determining the various steps for a ladder of exposure tasks, Tables 12 and 13 are two sample stepladders that might be suitable in helping Nathan to meet some of his goals (the eight-year-old boy described earlier). It might also help to refer back to his worry list outlined in Table 11 to see how the broad goals on the worry list have been transformed into more specific steps.

Rewards

I often find that rewards are the one area of an exposure program that parents and professionals tend to forget about. Sometimes it seems that the individual's efforts to practice exposure tasks are taken for granted as though the reduction in his anxiety as he learns to face his fears should be rewarding enough. But rewards are crucial! They are as critical a part of success in graded exposure tasks as any other step outlined in this chapter. I cannot emphasize enough how beneficial it can be to regularly reward the person for **all** attempts he makes to engage in an exposure task. Everyone benefits from a motivator for their efforts to tackle a task that is challenging. Therefore, if the person is practicing his exposure tasks five to seven times each week, then he needs to be rewarded each of those five to seven times for his success in the attempt. As discussed above, it is not easy for a person to experience initial discomfort by facing a fear. Therefore, rewards are critical in helping to motivate the person to persist with the exposure tasks and ultimately benefit from them.

Since the use of rewards is such a critical part of motivating the person to face his fears, it is important that you clarify with him, ahead of conducting the exposure task, exactly what the rewards will be. Negotiate rewards with the person. Just as it is beneficial to include the person in setting up stepladders and preparing for his exposure tasks, it is equally motivating to include him in choosing the rewards he will receive for his efforts. Sometimes you will also need to negotiate appropriate rewards with other team members, i.e., parents and teachers

Table 12 | Sample Stepladder for Fear of Speaking in Public

Goal: Giving a presentation at a school assembly

Step #	Description of task	Worry rating (out of 10)	Reward
1	Prepare my presentation	3	Twenty class points
2	Show my work on the presentation to the teacher	4	Choose the story time book in class
3	Answer a question aloud in class	5	Five minutes free time in class
4	Ask a question aloud during group discussion in class	5	Special after school treat with Mom
5	Read aloud in class	6	Go to the park after school
6	Practice my presentation in front of my family	6	Chore-free night at home
7	Share news with the class	7	A sticker sheet from the teacher
8	Practice reading my presentation in front of the teacher	7	A school award signed by the principal
9	Practice reading my presentation in front of the class	8	A treat from the school cafeteria
10	Practice the presentation, without my notes, in front of the class, while my classmates deliberately make funny faces at me	9	A new book
11	Practice the presentation, without my notes, in front of the class and deliberately make a mistake	9	Extra pocket money
12	Give the presentation at assembly	10	A camping trip with Dad

Table 13	Sample Stepladder for Fear of Birds			
Goal: Playing with my cousin's pet canary			
Step #	Description of task	Worry rating (out of 10)	Reward
1	Read about birds	2	A walk with Dad
2	Watch video footage of birds on the Internet	3	Choose a TV show to watch with Mom
3	Visit a pet shop and stand outside watching the birds in their cages	4	Choose what's for dinner
4	Go to the park and watch the birds	4	A bubble bath
5	Feed my cousin's pet canary when it is in its cage	5	Extra time on the computer
6	Stand in my cousin's room when he lets the canary out of its cage	6	Stay up thirty minutes later
7	Feed the canary out of the cage while my cousin holds it	7	Order take-out food for dinner
8	Pat my cousin's pet canary while my cousin holds it	8	A new movie on DVD
9	Hold and pat my cousin's pet canary without help	9	A new toy
10	Let my cousin's canary land on my shoulder and "kiss" me while I pat its chest	10	Mom or Dad take me to a movie with a friend and have dinner afterward

if the exposure task is happening at school (see Table 12). Examples of rewards are provided in Tables 12 and 13 to show how you might match rewards to the level of challenge of the task.

Of course, it stands to reason that punishments or negative consequences (e.g., removing a privilege such as computer time) would never be used if someone did not complete or cooperate with an exposure task. The idea is to set small enough steps for exposure (as in the examples provided in Tables 12 and 13) so that the person is set up to succeed—not feel overwhelmed by the task and, therefore, unable to complete it.

> ## Tips:
> 1. Rewards do not have to cost a lot of money.
> 2. The best type of reward for an individual, especially a child, is time with a parent (e.g., reading a book together, listening to music together, going for a walk together, playing together, or simply sitting alongside him and observing him while he plays on his own if he is more significantly affected by autism and prefers this).
> 3. Other rewards might include staying up later, choosing what's for dinner, a special dessert, extra time engaging in a preferred activity (e.g., computer time).
> 4. Bigger rewards such as toys, pocket money, special outings (e.g., going to the movies) are also reasonable. However, save them for more challenging exposure tasks that relate to steps further up the ladder.

4. Conduct the Exposure Tasks According to the Order Outlined on the Stepladder.

Following these additional tips for conducting exposure tasks may help you:

- Exposure occurs when the "real" situation (as outlined by the stepladder) is actually faced. Therefore, preparation must be done before conducting any exposure task. Preparation can include walking your child or client through the process of imagining the object or event, role playing the event together to practice what will happen and having a pretend "run through," and implementing other anxiety reducing strategies including relaxation and brave thinking.
- For people with autism, I have found it helpful to prepare a worksheet for each exposure task to cover the following sections:
  - ❑ what the task is;
  - ❑ how often the task will be attempted;
  - ❑ how long the task will last;
  - ❑ what type of preparation will occur before the exposure task, for example role playing, a practice

run through with an adult, reading a list of brave thoughts, doing a deep breathing exercise; and
- ❏ what reward(s) the person will receive.

- You can use separate headings and spaces to cover each of the sections listed above. It is a good idea to do this in consultation with the individual so that he takes more ownership of the task rather than to simply present it to him already completed, giving him a more passive role. When completing the worksheet with him, you can write down his ideas for him if he does not wish to write. If he benefits from visual supports, then you can use more pictures than words, i.e., pictures of the task, a picture of a calendar to mark when he will attempt the task, a picture of the type of preparation he will do (e.g., a picture of someone doing controlled breathing), and a picture of the reward he will receive. Essentially, what you are trying to do is ensure that the person fully understands the task and knows exactly what he needs to do to prepare for and complete the exposure task.

- During an exposure task, the person must stay in the situation long enough for his anxiety level to reduce. But how do you judge this? Perhaps one way to determine whether or not the person has stayed in the anxiety-provoking situation for long enough is to use a worry rating scale or a thermometer, as described earlier in this chapter. For example, you might decide that the person needs to stay in the situation until his worry level drops down to a rating of two on the scale. Regardless of whether or not you use a scale, the most important thing is that the person stays in the anxiety-provoking situation long enough to learn that he can cope; that the object or situation he fears is, in fact, safe; and that what he fears either does not occur or, if it does, is not as bad as he originally believed it to be.

- Each exposure task is practiced and repeated until it no longer produces excessive fear.

- Regular practice is essential! Typically, someone with an anxiety disorder has fears that have been present for a long time, sometimes years. Only practicing a task once or twice is not sufficient to properly overcome the fear. Daily practice is recommended, i.e., five to seven attempts each week.

- Be aware of any subtle tactics the person might use to avoid the feared object or situation. For example, some children will ask their parent to complete the exposure task with them because this helps them to feel better about the task. Others might try to cover their ears or eyes to avoid full confrontation with the feared object or situation. It is important to discourage avoidance. Remind them of their helpful thoughts or relaxation skills. It is okay to complete relaxation skills with them or to make suggestions for helpful thoughts they can remember if they are feeling nervous about the task. But, you need to be clear that they, alone, must fully experience the feared situation, without extra help or subtle attempts to avoid it. We do not want the person to avoid experiencing the full extent of his fear. In other words, you want the person to learn to attribute any reduction in his fear to his own bravery and the lack of "danger" he is noticing as he conducts the exposure tasks. We do not want the person to attribute reductions in his anxiety to some other factor such as the presence of another person for support and safety.

- Sometimes people might be fearful of an object or situation that causes pain (e.g., injections or shots, having blood taken, or going to the dentist). Essentially, the steps involved in helping them overcome their fear of these situations would be the same as described above. Again, the important thing to remember is that the steps on the ladders you prepare are small enough to be manageable—not so overwhelming that they cannot be achieved. For example, if you were tackling the fear of going to the dentist, then a first step of having the child's teeth cleaned at the dentist would be too challenging, whereas looking at pictures of a dental procedure might be more manageable.

- In addition, you need to pay particular attention to the kind of brave thoughts you work on with the person to ensure that they are realistic. For example, a thought such as "it won't hurt me" will not be helpful as it is not true. Rather, thoughts such as "It only lasts a few seconds. I've had a filling before and survived so I can do it again. It won't hurt as much as when I accidently scraped my knee at school, and I was brave then" might be appropriate.

- Apart from relaxation skills, you can also employ tools to help the person distract himself from the pain during the procedure, e.g., ask him to imagine something that he enjoys, like a favorite vacation destination, allow him to listen to music during the procedure, or allow him to play a hand-held computer game during the procedure (if appropriate).

Putting it All Together

This chapter has outlined in detail each of the four main components involved in CBT for anxious people with an ASD and related strategies. What does it look like for a client when we put all the components together? Below is a case example to demonstrate.

CBT Case example: Felix, a six-year-old boy with high functioning autism

Felix's parents came to see me because Felix was having difficulty coping with losing and not being the first chosen at school for various activities. His school peers were reportedly becoming frustrated by his behavior and beginning to exclude him from the general play at recess and lunch time. In class, his peers were avoiding teaming up with him for group work. Consequently, Felix was feeling left out and isolated at school.

According to Felix's parents and his classroom teacher, Felix would become worried before lining up to enter or exit the classroom, before beginning a board game or sporting game with his classmates, and during any classes in which point or reward systems were used. Specifically, Felix wanted to be the first in line, the child who always won the game, or the person who earned the most points within the class. If he felt that he might be missing points or losing in a game, he would either try to falsify the results (e.g., pretend that he had earned a point when he hadn't) or would request commendations from his classroom teacher by asking, "What about my good listening in class? Do I get fifty house points?" If Felix did not win a game or receive the most notoriety in the classroom, he would cry or run out of the room. What typically followed was a group of teachers searching for him throughout the school grounds and then cajoling him to come back to class once he was found.

Felix parents indicated that his worries about whether he was the "best" at an activity or the "winner" also affected his home life. The family was fearful of playing board games or other turn-taking games with him at home in case he lost and could not cope with the outcome. They reported that during games he would try to regularly check who was winning and would become visibly upset if he felt that he was not winning.

Following school observations of Felix and a detailed assessment with him and his family at the clinic, we determined that Felix was worried that losing meant he was "stupid" or "a loser." He reported that he worried about this each time he played a game or each time a reward system was used in the classroom. From observations, and teacher and parent reports, it seemed that Felix was able to work himself up into a state of panic about winning or being "the best." Felix, himself, reported nausea and headaches during lessons when point systems were used.

Felix's CBT intervention involved four components. First, time was spent educating him about feelings including specific feelings of worry or fear. He completed "mind reading" games working on identifying emotions in himself and others as well as role plays to help clearly demonstrate his emotional responses. For specific education about anxiety, it was explained to Felix that his worries were getting in the way of him having fun at school and at home and, therefore, he needed to learn how to "boss them away" rather than let them take control and make him sad. Worksheets and puppet characters were used to help Felix learn about the way in which worry can cause problems and stop us from having fun. Felix and his parents were also given visual diaries to keep track of when his worries were causing him problems at school and at home. A reward system was used to reinforce Felix's participation in his homework tasks.

Second, Felix was taught controlled breathing skills. Colored mats were set up in the classroom and in his room at home to visually mark the "spots" where Felix could practice his breathing skills. Again, visual diaries were used to help monitor his practice with reward systems used to acknowledge Felix's efforts in practicing breathing regularly. Felix's parents and classroom teacher were given palm-sized cards that displayed pictorially the steps involved in the controlled breathing procedure. The cards were placed next to the colored mats in the classroom and at home.

There was also a card for Felix to keep in his pocket at school so that he could readily and independently follow the listed steps involved in completing his breathing skills.

Third, puppets and worksheets were used to teach Felix about worries and helpful thoughts. He was also given written and illustrated lists of examples of unhelpful and helpful thoughts rather than having to generate his own. In part, this was done because he struggled with reading, but, also, to make the task less intellectually demanding. The lists were used when discussing the puppet's thinking and reactions in various anxiety-provoking situations. For example, if a puppet acted worried when it was about to complete a spelling test, Felix was instructed to use the thoughts lists to try to determine what kind of worrying thought the puppet might be experiencing. Similarly, Felix was then taught to use the brave thoughts list to find a better thought for the puppet to use. The puppet was then used to demonstrate the same process in relation to situations regarding winning and losing or earning the most points in the classroom so that Felix could observe and discuss the puppet's behavior regarding situations that Felix also worried about.

A "brave thoughts" book was then developed for Felix and the puppet to use whenever Felix was worried about winning, being "the best," or "looking stupid." Thoughts in the book were kept simple and included "Everyone has turns at losing a game," "Losing doesn't mean I am stupid," "Losing can help me see how to play better next time," and "I am still a good student, even if I am not picked to line up first."

A visual choice board was also put in place in the classroom so that when Felix became anxious, he could be referred to the choice board to pick an option from a range of pictorially presented choices for how to calm down including: take a break to do breathing exercises on the special mat, read my "brave thoughts" book, talk to the teacher about how I'm feeling, and think of my favorite food to eat and imagine eating it.

Fourth, a stepladder was set up in consultation with Felix and his parents targeting winning/losing. Initial steps on the ladder included going down one ladder in the game of Chutes and Ladders. Steps further up the ladder included refraining from asking about points in class or about being first in line. Steps toward the top end of the ladder included deliberately letting someone win a game (e.g., a tennis game or board game). Reward systems were used to help motivate Felix at each step on his ladder. Felix was given a new worksheet in preparation for each exposure task to ensure that role plays were conducted ahead of "real life" exposure, that Felix had a suitable list of brave thoughts to use to combat worries in each exposure activity, and that Felix knew when to practice his breathing skills.

Felix, his parents, and his classroom teacher have all reported that there has been a reduction in Felix's anxiety and his challenging behavior regarding winning/losing and being "the best." According to Felix's parents, he is now able to play board games at home, lose the game, and cope. Moreover, Felix has reported having more fun at school because he is better able to join in and socialize with his peers. Felix no longer avoids games with his peers in case he might lose. Moreover, because he is learning how to be a "better sport," he no longer displays challenging behavior that, in the past, would have caused his peers frustration and reduced their desire to play with him.

What Other Considerations Need to Be Made for CBT Programs for People with Autism?

When using CBT, essentially, there are five key considerations that I believe we need to account for to ensure the best possible improvements in our children, students, or clients with an ASD.

1. Visual Supports

When possible, it is beneficial to include visual supports within CBT programs. For example, worksheets, visual checklists, or visual work systems could be used to teach children the key steps involved in relaxation skills. Using checklists encourages the person to follow a step-by-step guide. Therefore, it helps ensure that the person takes ownership and responsibility for noting when he has completed each relevant step of a breathing or muscle relaxation exercise. For nonreaders or early readers, checklists might need to be pictorial and interactive. For example, individual steps involved in a breathing exercise could be displayed using pictures with each picture in the sequence attached separately to a board with Velcro®. The person could then be responsible for moving the picture off the board as he completes each step until at the end of the breathing or relaxation exercise, the board is empty to show that the person has finished the exercise. (See Appendix C for books that provide more information on visual supports.)

Visual schedules and time tables might also be helpful to display and keep track of practice requirements in a CBT program. For example, visual schedules might need to be included to help people develop clear and regular time slots for practicing relaxation skills or exposure exercises.

2. Scripts, Lists, and Social Stories

In general, CBT programs for typically developing anxious people use few visual supports and rely heavily on the person completing cognitive tasks without extra visual cues or prompts. The underlying assumption is that typically developing adolescents are able to analyze their own thinking style and have the more fluid thinking and better developed executive functioning skills to look for patterns in their reasoning. Therefore, cognitive therapy in a CBT program for typically developing teenagers might involve asking people to:

- list recent unhelpful thoughts that made them feel anxious;
- consider the style or type of unhelpful thought it was, i.e., overgeneralizing (e.g., "That person didn't laugh at my joke; everyone must think I'm boring"), catastrophizing (e.g., I think I made a mistake in answering that math question. I'll probably fail the math exam and have to repeat the year"), black and white thinking (e.g., "If I'm not the best at tennis, then there's no point playing"), personalizing (e.g., "John seemed a bit down today, it was probably my fault because of something I said to him");
- look for evidence or facts to show that the unhelpful thought or worry might not be true or as "bad" as they initially believed; and
- develop an alternative, more helpful or braver thought to use instead.

However, for people with an ASD, the above listed steps might be too abstract, particularly in light of their relatively weaker planning, organization, and problem solving skills. Indeed, such complex tasks might even be unnecessary for a person with an ASD whose thinking style tends to be more black and white, rule-based, and rigid than fluid and abstract. Therefore, for a person with an ASD, it might be better to keep it simple in the cognitive component of a CBT program.

Using scripts or stories that show characters or individuals who might experience similar worries to the person with an ASD helps to provide a more concrete framework to highlight the difference between worries and brave thoughts. It is always easier to recognize examples of worried thinking in another person than it is to recall your own.

Lists of unhelpful and helpful thoughts allow people with an ASD to quickly pick from the listed alternatives the ones that apply to them. Again, this simpler cognitive exercise saves the extra effort and difficulty of having to generate their own examples. If there is enough variety in the types of helpful and unhelpful thoughts listed, then the people with ASD are bound to recognize a thought that they can relate to or will find helpful. Moreover, in the intensity of the moment when a person feels anxious, it might be much easier for the person with an ASD to refer to an already prepared list of helpful thoughts, than to try to work out without a visual cue what brave thoughts to generate.

Following this logic, social stories or simple visual checklists might be beneficial in CBT programs for anxious people with autism. Step by step stories or notes regarding what to do when anxious provide a concrete "plan of attack" against worries so that people do not feel lost when they actually face an anxiety provoking object or activity. Plans such as the following are more likely to be beneficial for someone with an ASD than "thinking on the spot" when he is anxious:

Step 1: Stop and take some deep breaths until my body feels less worried.

Step 2: Check my brave thoughts list.

Step 3: Pick a thought and read it aloud (or say it to myself).

Step 4: Have another try.

3. Cognitive Challenging for People Who Have High Support Needs

Cognitive therapy tasks might be too complicated for people who have an ASD and associated intellectual delay. If even simplified cognitive exercises as described above are too difficult, then the cognitive component can be dropped altogether. Instead, more emphasis and time can be spent on teaching and practicing relaxation skills and setting up graded exposure tasks.

With regard to exposure tasks, the assumption for anxious individuals is that by repeatedly facing a feared object or activity, they will get used to the object or situation without needing to learn extra cognitive restructuring skills. However, for people with high support needs, more emphasis might need to be placed on making exposure tasks very concrete using visual sequences, schedules, and token systems for rewards. An example could be to use photos to show a visual sequence of the person facing his feared situation then being rewarded instantly for his efforts. Repeating such sequences until they are well learned and the person eventually desensitizes is still essential.

4. Adequate Time for Skill Generalization

People with an ASD tend to have difficulty learning skills and generalizing those learned skills from one situation or environment to another. Therefore, more time needs to be taken to teach the respective components and skills of a CBT program. In a CBT program for people without autism, relaxation skills might be taught in one session; however, for people with an ASD, many sessions might be required to learn the skills involved. Moreover, extra time might be required to help people learn to generalize their use of relaxation skills across several settings where they tend to be anxious.

5. Social Skills

Children who are socially anxious (regardless of whether or not they have an ASD) tend to have some social skill difficulties. We know that they can feel less confident in using their skills for fear of "getting it wrong" or looking foolish. However, it is also possible that they have weaker social skills because they avoid social situations so much that they fall out of practice.

For people with autism, social skills deficits are part of their core difficulties. Therefore, their social anxiety is likely to be even greater than what we would observe in other anxious children who do not have an ASD. Consequently, it is very important that anxiety support for a person with autism also involves some element of social skills training either with the person himself or via work with his parents. This training can occur before starting a CBT program or it might be incorporated as a separate module in an anxiety intervention program. Regardless, it is very important that social skills are taught. Specifically, it is important to cover a range of social skills including:

- the use of appropriate gestures, body language, facial expression, and posture;
- appropriate tone, volume, and rate of speech;
- initial conversation skills such as the use of open-ended questions, offering personal information, asking questions about other's interests, thoughts, or feelings;
- friendship skills such as joining in on the playground, sharing, turn-taking, giving positive feedback to friends to show your enjoyment; and
- assertiveness such as asking for help in class or on the playground and responding appropriately to any teasing or bullying that might occur.

Is a CBT Program the Best Option for All Anxious People with an ASD?

CBT-based anxiety intervention targets individuals whose fears or worries are based on irrational or catastrophic thinking in the absence of actual evidence to prove the fear is founded. For example, if I worried about talking to other people for fear of making a mistake or someone laughing at me when generally I have no real difficulties communicating with other people, then my thinking would be considered irrational and my worries unfounded. In this example, a CBT program that uses cognitive restructuring and exposure to target my fears about talking to other people might be appropriate. However, for people with autism, it can be argued that sometimes their anxiety is exacerbated because of "real" evidence that supports their worries (Wood et al., 2009). For example, a person with autism who worries about socializing might have actual evidence to show that he is genuinely not socially successful, particularly given that poor social skills are a core deficit of autism. Similarly, a person who is anxious about his ability to perform certain self-care tasks might have actual evidence to show that he is not yet competent in toileting, dressing, or organizing his own daily routine. Again, limitations in daily living skills are well documented for people with autism (e.g., Klin et al., 2007). In both of the above examples, it would be hard to try to convince the person that his worries are unfounded. Therefore, a CBT program that targets worry might not be the appropriate starting point for intervention for that person. Rather, a social skills or adaptive living skills program that teaches the person how to socialize more effectively or better manage his daily living activities might be the best way to help him worry less and develop more self-confidence.

In summary, the following rule of thumb might be helpful in determining when CBT is the best treatment to use. First, consider whether the person's anxiety is based on rational or irrational thinking. If the person genuinely lacks skills and feels anxious about a skills deficit, then it is skill development that he needs, i.e., a social skills group or individual social skills training. This should occur before any exposure tasks are set up so that he is not engaging in exposure that displays his skill deficits and makes him even more anxious. After he develops better social and daily living skills, if anxiety around these issues still exists, then a CBT-based intervention might be in order. However, if a person's fears are unfounded (i.e., he does not actually lack skills, rather he falsely believes that there is something to fear), then CBT as the first point of intervention might be a good approach to adopt.

As noted in Chapter 7, sometimes medication is used to help reduce and manage anxiety symptoms. At times, anxiety can be so severe that there is no point beginning a CBT-based intervention until the person has shown some reduction in his symptoms through the use of anti-anxiety medication.

There are some occasions when it is not sensible to use a CBT-based intervention. If time does not permit your spending a few hours each week working on addressing anxiety difficulties in your child, student, or client, then a CBT-based intervention is not really recommended. Similarly, if you are working with someone who has no motivation to address his own anxiety difficulties, then you might find that CBT is not the best approach for that person, given that CBT focuses on teaching the person skills to ultimately help him become more independent in overcoming his anxiety.

In Summary

- CBT seems to be a promising treatment for anxiety difficulties for individuals with autism, particularly people with high functioning autism or Asperger's disorder.

- CBT involves four key components:
  1. Education about feelings of worry or anxiety in order to help people develop better awareness of when they are feeling anxious and, therefore, when to implement skills to combat their anxiety.
  2. Relaxation skills to combat the physiological symptoms of anxiety.
  3. Cognitive restructuring skills to help shift unhelpful worries into more realistic or brave ways of thinking about a situation.
  4. Graded exposure to help target avoidance of anxiety-provoking situations and, in turn, allow people to learn that they are capable of remaining in an anxiety provoking situation without any "danger."
- When using a CBT program with a person with autism, it is important to ensure that some considerations are made including:
  - Using visual supports for skills checklists and practice schedules.
  - Using scripts, checklists, and social stories to teach and prompt helpful or brave thinking.
  - For people with very high support needs, omitting the cognitive challenging component all together and focusing instead on relaxation skills and graded exposure tasks.
  - Allowing more time to teach each skill so that generalization occurs.
  - Ensuring that social skills are taught either before beginning the CBT intervention or as a part of it.
- CBT intervention is not necessarily the best first option for all people with autism who are anxious. Before beginning a CBT program that targets anxiety, it is first essential to determine whether or not the anxiety is based on genuine skill deficits or unfounded worries.

9 | Treating Anxiety in Parents and Siblings of People with Autism

The Turner Family

After attending a school consultation for Mark, a six-year-old boy with high functioning autism, his mother approached me and asked if I'd be willing to meet with her other son, Bradley, a nine-year-old who is typically developing. Mrs. Turner expressed concerns about the level of stress and anxiety in the household because of the challenges of living with Mark. She was worried that Bradley was not coping with Mark and that he was building up an intense dislike toward him. She said that the two boys often ended up in fist fights with each other at home. Mrs. Turner reported that Bradley seemed to be becoming more and more withdrawn at home and his relationship with her, especially, was strained. She said she wondered whether Bradley was feeling rejected because of all the time required of her to manage Mark's therapy and learning support. She also reported that Bradley was making statements like, "I wish I was an only child. Will things ever get better for Mark? Will Mark ever have friends or will he be lonely? Will life at home always be this hard? Will you guys always have to spend so much time with Mark? Will Mark ever be normal?" Bradley was experiencing mixed emotions towards Mark and the family including frustration with Mark and the challenges of living with him. Also he was worrying about Mark's future and his own future and happiness.

Beyond the challenges of living with a son with autism, Mrs. Turner spoke of her own anxiety and described herself as a "worrier." She said that she frequently felt worried about many issues, including the success of her business, her relationships, her ability to be a good parent, the children's health, their futures, e.g., post-high school options (even though both boys were only in elementary school), her ability to manage home affairs and routines, and most recently, whether or not she was adopting the right path of intervention for Mark following his recent diagnosis of anxiety.

When I met with Bradley, he seemed as though he was nine going on nineteen. His maturity and insight were incredible. He easily identified and could discuss at length a range of worries that he experienced about Mark and the family. He said he felt worried that life was going to be difficult all the time because of Mark and the tantrums he had at home. Bradley talked at length about feeling as though he was expected to put up with "more than a nine-year-old should have to" in terms of "letting Mark have his way." He felt confused and worried about whether to "give in" to Mark to prevent Mark's frustration and challenging behavior and avoid extra stress on his parents, or whether to push for what he, himself, wanted. For example, he talked about playing Mark's favorite board games and card games and feeling confused as to whether to let Mark win so he wouldn't have a tantrum, which would stress out his parents, or whether to play "normally" and potentially win the game.

Bradley also described feeling worried about his relationship with his parents, especially his mother. He said he thought she was spending more time with Mark "because of the autism" and he felt as though he was always being left to "sort himself out."

The Turner family is not unique. Many siblings and parents I see have the same worries and frustrations as Bradley and his mother. Although the focus of this book is about anxiety in people with autism and how to manage it, it is important not to forget the broader family unit. As we can see from Bradley and Mrs. Turner's descriptions, often, there is significant anxiety within other family members that, if left unaddressed, can cause problems for the whole family unit.

Parent Anxiety

Since anxiety-related difficulties have a documented negative impact on families of typically developing children (Anderson, 1994; Keller, Lavoir, Wunder, Beardslee, Schwarts & Roth, 1992; Messer & Beidel, 1994), it is not a stretch to assume that caring for a child with both autism and associated anxiety will result in even greater distress for those families. Studies comparing parents of typically developing children with parents of children with an ASD demonstrate that the latter tend to have fewer coping resources (Sivberg, 2002; Fombonne et al., 2001) and higher rates of anxiety and/or depression (Fombonne et al., 2001; Piven et al., 1991; Wolf, Noh, Fisman & Speechly, 1989). Therefore, it might be hypothesized that parents of children with both an ASD and an anxiety disorder might have even fewer coping resources than parents of children with an ASD but without an anxiety disorder.

We also know from research that children with anxiety difficulties tend to live in families where the parents themselves also experience anxiety (van der Bruggen, Stams & Bögels, 2008). This notion that often parents model anxious behavior for their children was discussed in Chapter 4. So, apart from employing the parenting strategies discussed in Chapter 5 to help encourage bravery and reduce anxiety in a child, it is essential that parents or siblings who are anxious get support in managing their own anxiety difficulties.

Just like in the example of Mrs. Turner, many parents I work with indicate that they were anxious long before they had a child with autism. Often, when discussing their family histories, parents will state that before starting a family, they experienced some history of anxiety difficulties such as panic attacks, performance anxiety while studying, a tendency to be perfectionistic, or a general tendency to worry. If a parent already has a history of anxiety and then has a child with autism, it is possible that the parent is going to be at risk of experiencing an anxiety disorder herself. Consequently, professionals working with such parents need to consider referring parents for their own individual support to manage their own anxiety difficulties.

How Do You Support an Anxious Parent?

Relaxation Skills

The relaxation skills discussed in Chapter 8 are certainly suitable for anxious people of any age, including parents. Although parents may supervise their child's relaxation skills practice, or even participate in the activity with their child, it is important that anxious parents set time aside to conduct controlled breathing or progressive muscle relaxation (PMR) practice by and for themselves. Just as the person with autism will best learn the skill by engaging in regular practice times separate from using relaxation in the moments when she feels anxious, so too will parents. Although parents might not need to set up practice charts or diaries to monitor their own relaxation practice, the following are useful suggestions for ensuring that practice occurs:

- Program your smart phone to remind you of set practice times. When the alarm goes off, take a few minutes to conduct your controlled breathing practice.
- Put a reminder note such as "five minutes breathing practice" or "ten minutes muscle relaxation" on your computer as a screensaver.
- Alternatively, program the reminder note to your computer organizer program.
- Set five to ten minutes aside during your work lunch break to do some relaxation.
- Stick a reminder note on your bathroom mirror so that whenever you use the bathroom, you can take an extra minute or so to do some controlled breathing.
- Set aside time for at least four progressive muscle relaxation (PMR) practice sessions each week. Pick a consistent time and try stick to it just as you would with other activities such as using the gym, walking the dog, or preparing meals.
- Let your spouse or partner, a family member, or close friend know that you are working on some relaxation skills to help reduce anxiety and ask them to check in with you each week to see how your practice is going. Sometimes the extra "pressure" of someone else knowing you are working toward a goal can help you stick to it more vigilantly.

Individual Therapy

For some parents, their anxiety is so impairing that they need to seek assistance from a mental health professional. There is nothing to be ashamed of in seeking help. Indeed, it is always better to err on the side of getting extra support than to go without it altogether. A mental health professional (e.g., a clinical psychologist) is typically a good professional to seek out if your anxiety is affecting your daily living. The following are some signs that should prompt you to seek extra help:

- If you are experiencing regular (e.g., daily) physical anxiety symptoms such as nausea, diarrhea, muscle tension, headaches, etc.
- If you are experiencing regular panic attacks
- If you are unable to sleep because of worry or anxiety
- If you have lost your appetite because of worry or anxiety
- If you cannot concentrate or adequately complete daily tasks because of worry or anxiety
- If you regularly use alcohol or some other substance to relax

Again, since we know that parents can inadvertently model anxious behavior for their children, then any attempts you make to support your child's anxiety via treatment or the intervention strategies outlined in this book might ultimately be undermined if your own anxiety remains "out of check." Conversely, if you make efforts to get your own anxiety under control, you are setting a positive example for your child and modeling good anxiety "hygiene" for her.

Parent Support Groups

Groups where parents can meet to exchange information and discuss with other parents their experiences of raising children with autism might indirectly reduce parental anxiety. Parents find it reassuring to meet other parents who have had similar experiences and know what it is like to raise a child with autism. Some groups are highly structured, offering regular meeting times with topics and related advice for each meeting, for example schooling options, toilet training, and social skills. Other groups are more informal, providing a network of parents who simply spend time together as a social outlet, which, in turn, can help reduce anxiety. Regardless of the level of structure, it is important for anxious parents to have some sense that their worries are "normal" and that many other parents have coped with similar concerns in the lives. For example, during an anxiety management group that I ran last year for parents whose children attended a special school, it became clear that many parents in the group were reassured by phrases such as "Yes, that happened to us too," or "We had that problem for years and in the end this is what worked for us...."

In Sydney, Autism Spectrum Australia (the national nonprofit body specializing in services for people with autism and their families) runs a great program called "Someone to Turn to." Essentially, parents seeking support are linked with other "mentor" parents who have children with similar levels of functioning. The "mentor" parents become a point of contact for the parents seeking support if they wish to discuss concerns regarding difficulties they are experiencing with their child or are simply looking for some reassurance. It is an excellent initiative.

One word of caution regarding support groups and forums is to be careful not to take all information provided in them as the "gospel truth." Naturally, each parent's experience of raising a child with autism is different. Therefore, what works for one parent might not work for another. For example, forums or parent organizations where parents insist that certain intervention methods (e.g., strict diets) are the only way to "cure" a child with autism are unhelpful and serve to increase other parents' anxiety rather than reduce it. The best advice that I can give in this regard would be to choose interventions that fit your child's individual strengths and weaknesses. There is no single treatment for autism. Rather, interventions need to be chosen according to how they address the various strengths or difficulties of each person. The value of a good parent support group is that other parents can tell you about the pros and cons of their own intervention choices and broader experiences rather than dictate exactly which path you should follow.

Time for Yourself

Given the demands of caring for a person with special needs, it is certainly understandable that many parents do not allocate time for themselves. Between managing therapy appointments, schooling, extra-curricular activities, the needs and schedules of other children in the family, and the daily life activities that are part of running a household, there is not usually much left over. However, if you are an anxious parent, it is essential that you set aside time for yourself. The less time that is allocated to oneself, the more likely an anxious parent is to become consumed by her worries because she has no distractions from the situations that trigger her anxiety. Time for oneself does not have to be as time consuming as a weekend away or as desperate as locking yourself away from the family! It can be as simple as ten minutes reading a book or walking to the park and back. The simpler the activity, the easier it will be to include it in your daily life and the less overwhelming it will be to make time for. Some ideas include:

- A phone call to a favorite friend or relative
- Making yourself a cup of tea, coffee, or hot chocolate
- Reading the paper for ten minutes
- A quick walk
- Listening to a favorite piece of music
- Going to the gym or another form of exercise
- Preparing a favorite meal or even reading a new recipe
- Ten minutes planning some aspect of the next family vacation
- Gardening
- Shopping (even online)

Remember What is "Normal"

Sometimes I work with parents who micro-manage their child's development. That is, they seem to worry about every aspect of their child's development to the point where they overlook what might actually be considered "normal" in terms of the way their child behaves. It is natural for parents of a child with special needs to want to protect their child and ensure that she is developing to meet her full potential. However, it is important to bear in mind that sometimes the behaviors we observe in people with autism can occur just as frequently in other people their age and are absolutely appropriate in terms of what we would expect of "normal" development. An example from a parent I work with springs to mind:

Valerie

Sally is a seventeen-year-old-girl with Asperger's disorder. Her mother, Valerie, is highly anxious. Sally has a history of difficulty with organization as is often the case for people her age who have an autism spectrum disorder. Valerie worries constantly about Sally's homework, her ability to manage her time with assignments, and her ability to study adequately for school exams. One weekend last year, Valerie sent me a three-page email complaining about Sally's behavior and seeking an urgent appointment with myself and Sally. According to Valerie, Sally had two assignments and a home science project to complete, plus three exams to study for. Valerie reported that when she tried to assist Sally by organizing a timetable for her and telling her what to study or work on,

Sally became frustrated, yelling at her mother, stating that she wanted to be left alone. Consequently, Valerie wrote to me wondering whether or not Sally needed some individual assistance for "emotion regulation difficulties." She also queried whether this kind of behavior might be a precursor to more aggressive behavior or anger-management difficulties and depression if it was left unchecked.

When I spoke to Valerie the following Monday, I informed her that an urgent appointment would not be necessary and that it was highly unlikely that Sally was at risk of becoming aggressive or depressed on the basis of an incident like the one Valerie described. When Valerie asked why, I suggested that she try to recall her own adolescence and a time when she had a heavy workload at high school (e.g., end of year exams). I then asked Valerie whether or not she recalled feeling overwhelmed by her heavy workload. She acknowledged that she often felt overwhelmed. Finally, I asked Valerie whether or not she might have yelled at a parent who was telling her how to do her work or study for an exam during a time of high stress. Valerie fell silent. Eventually, Valerie said, "I guess we can wait to see you at our regularly scheduled appointment instead of coming in sooner."

In this example, Sally's mother had lost sight of the fact that it is very "normal" for an adolescent (whether she has autism or not) to find parental directions about work completion slightly intrusive and overbearing when she is stressed out by a heavy workload. The last thing that any person feels like listening to when she knows she has a lot of work to do is a parent that might come across as though she is nagging. But because of Sally's diagnosis, Valerie seemed to overlook that her daughter's behavior might actually be "normal." Rather, she thought instantly that this was another of Sally's problems that needed "fixing."

As a general rule, I recommend that parents regularly ask themselves whether what they are worrying about seems "normal" or not. How can you judge "normal"? Perhaps consider what other non-autistic children might do in similar circumstances. Alternatively, as was suggested to Valerie in the example above, try to reflect on your own behavior at a similar stage of development as your son or daughter. If you feel that you were probably behaving in the same way and you currently see other kids without autism behaving in this way, then that is usually a good indication that you might be "over-worrying."

CBT for Anxious Parents

Given the promising results of using CBT to treat anxiety, it seems reasonable to argue that CBT might be a suitable treatment option for anxious parents of people with an ASD. Essentially, the four key components of CBT would remain the same. Differences might relate more to the content of worries being addressed than the skills taught. For example, in a CBT program for anxious parents, the structure and focus might look something like this:

- Education about Anxiety:
  - Detailed explanations regarding the core symptoms of anxiety
  - Explanations regarding the difference between helpful and unhelpful levels of anxiety
  - Tasks to help learn how to recognize and monitor anxiety (e.g., diaries)
  - Education regarding the role of avoidance in maintaining anxiety
  - Information regarding direct and indirect ways that parents might avoid what makes them anxious (e.g., checking behaviors, seeking reassurance, choosing not to complete or participate in certain activities)

- Relaxation Skills:
  - Controlled breathing
  - Progressive Muscle Relaxation exercises with an emphasis on how to use PMR to manage general stress and tension
  - Using visual imagery as a means of relaxing (e.g., recalling a favorite vacation destination or mentally walking through eating a favorite meal)

- Cognitive Restructuring
  - Teaching parents about the way that thinking affects our feelings
  - Teaching parents how to monitor their own anxious thinking (e.g., using diaries or daily record sheets)
  - Teaching parents techniques to find evidence against their own unhelpful or "faulty" thoughts (e.g.,

testing out their hypotheses like running an experiment, recalling what has happened in past experiences, searching for facts to support or refute their worried thoughts, reducing unrealistic expectations they might have of themselves by asking them to research or interview people they admire or respect and find examples of when such people have had similar problems or made similar mistakes)
- ❑ Challenging unrealistic thoughts that parents might report they have about themselves, e.g. they are not good enough, they could be doing a better job supporting their child with autism, by now their child with autism should be progressing further, they need to "cure" their child, their child will never be as happy as other people

- ■ Graded Exposure
  - ❑ Developing stepladders that address a parent's own worries rather than her child's worries

    For example, a parent who is a perfectionist, with daily unfounded worries about making mistakes in her work setting. Graded exposure tasks did not involve her child, rather, tasks centered on the parent deliberately making mistakes and dressing in a progressively unkempt style in the workplace in order to cope with the possibility of portraying an imperfect image to others.

What If a Parent is Highly Anxious But Won't Seek Help or Admit There is a Problem?

Perhaps the short answer to the above question is best summarized by the adage, "You can lead a horse to water but you can't make it drink!" Clearly, once someone is an adult, if she is adamant that she doesn't need support, then there is little that can be done to force it upon her.

Alternatively, if you are an anxious parent, you might not want to seek assistance in managing your own anxiety because you feel ashamed or feel that, in some way, it is a sign that you are unable to cope.

Moreover, you might feel concerned that in taking time to address your own anxiety difficulties, you are in some way detracting from time spent supporting your son or daughter with autism. These justifications are all understandable; however, as noted earlier, the longer you go without some form of support, the more likely this is to undermine success that your child may be having in her own intervention program.

If you are the partner of someone who is reluctant to seek help or a professional working with such a parent, then some of the following strategies might be useful:

- Gather data, i.e., keep a running record of how often you observe signs of anxiety in the person and discuss this with her.
- Give the person some information to take away and read regarding anxiety and how it manifests. Offer to make a time to discuss it with her if she would like to.
- If you are a clinician, then you might ask the parent to complete some self-report measures on anxiety in adults in order to show her where her reported levels of anxiety fall compared to what you might expect of other people in the population.
- Find examples of when the person's anxiety might be adversely affecting her child (e.g., if she is modeling anxious behavior) and try to discuss your observations with her.
- Consider offering the person a self-help anxiety guide or resources (e.g., "Mastering your Anxiety and Panic: Workbook," Barlow and Craske, 2007) rather than suggesting that she see a professional.
- Give the person a list of professionals to contact in her own time, as she sees fit.

Sibling Anxiety

It is often the case that siblings of children with an ASD are overlooked. Generally, parents do not deliberately choose to focus more on one child than another; however, caring for someone with autism usually involves allocating more time, support, and attention to that person than to her siblings.

Siblings of people with autism can be vulnerable to experiencing anxiety for several reasons. Less attention, time, or support allocated to them might result in them feeling insecure and lacking self-confidence. In addition, some siblings might take on the family pressures of living with a person with autism and worry about family circumstances, for example, if there is enough money to cover their brother's or sister's intervention costs and also allow the family to go on vacations from time to time. Other siblings can feel embarrassed or self-conscious because of their brother or sister with autism, i.e., feeling socially uncomfortable if they attend the same school as their sibling or worrying about whether people think there might also be something "wrong" with them if they have a sibling with special needs. Siblings can also worry about the person with autism. They might become anxious thinking about their brother's or sister's difficulties in making friends or learning at school. They might also place extra pressure on themselves to become like a third parent to the person with autism, for example by trying to help teach her how to make friends or how to complete academic tasks. Consider the example of one of my clients:

Alexandra and Her Family

When Alexandra's parents brought her to see me, they were concerned about her self-esteem and her tendency to be very anxious. Alexandra is ten years old. She is the eldest of five children with two very caring and supportive parents, Edith and Tim. Her brother Lucas, the second eldest in the family, has autism.

According to Edith and Tim, Alexandra always seems worried about something. They said she worries about the family income and how they will make ends meet. They report that when they go grocery shopping with her, she constantly worries about whether they can afford what they are purchasing, despite her parents informing her that they can. Edith and Tim also mentioned that Alexandra frequently asks about how Lucas is progressing with his therapy and whether he is going to be able to make friends when he gets to school next year. Alexandra also worries about her own school work. She is struggling with her reading and requires extra assistance from a tutor. Edith says that Alexandra worries about seeing the tutor because it costs money and may be taking money away from Lucas's therapy needs. Edith and Tim say that Alexandra frequently asks them if they are happy or whether they are worried about Lucas. She often volunteers to go over Lucas's therapy drills at home with him to help ensure that he is learning them effectively. At school, she is having difficulty making friends due to a lack of self-confidence.

Just like Bradley, when I met Alexandra, she presented like a mature adult, even though she was only ten years old. She talked as though she was a parent in the household, making frequent statements such as, "We are thinking of changing Lucas's therapy schedule" or "We are working on Lucas's play skills at the moment so that when we send him to school, it will be easier for him to know how to join in." In completing some self-report measures regarding anxiety and self-esteem, Alexandra seemed to confirm that she had many worries and was insecure in her own abilities to make friends and read.

Sessions with Alexandra focused on trying to shift her worried thoughts about the family and Lucas. In particular, we worked on cognitive restructuring skills such as teaching her to find evidence for and against her worries in order to develop more helpful cognitions.

Intervention also involved working with Edith and Tom to find ways to allocate more time and attention to Alexandra. We focused on looking for opportunities for them to reward and respond to "brave" behavior rather than spending time answering her questions when she was trying to discuss worries about the family budget or Lucas's treatment.

Moreover, we also focused on trying to redefine Alexandra's role within the family, that is to help her live her life more like a child and less like a third parent. Edith and Tim found special jobs that they could give Alexandra that were more age-appropriate, e.g., keeping the playroom tidy and making sure that the dinner table was set each night rather than discussing family finances, Lucas's therapy regime, and other parent responsibilities with her.

Social exposure tasks were also used to help Alexandra develop more confidence in her interactions with her peers at school. She was given practice tasks including talking to her peers, joining in play, and arranging play dates. All tasks were rewarded in terms of her bravery and confidence in carrying them out.

In general, Alexandra's example highlights the importance of tending to the self-esteem and self-confidence difficulties that are often present in siblings of a person with an ASD. The following strategies might assist you in this process:

- Teach the sibling ways to combat her own worried thoughts using brave thoughts and help her develop a brave thinking list or diary.
- Teach the sibling how to look for evidence to show that her worried thoughts might be false.

- Avoid responding to or reassuring her when she asks questions based on her worries in order to reduce anxiety. It is important for her to become more independent in reassuring herself rather than an adult doing it for her.
- Use graded exposure, as described in Chapter 8, to help the sibling face any fears or worries she might have regarding her own abilities.
- As parents, look for opportunities to praise and positively reinforce "bravery" and confidence frequently within the sibling.
- Allocate special roles within the household to the sibling and reward her independence and confidence in carrying out these roles.
- Allocate "worry time" to the sibling to discuss any pressures or worries she might be experiencing as well as to help her problem-solve ways to overcome her worries.
- Limit discussion of worries to "worry time" rather than responding to worry-based questions or statements at other times during the day.
- Ensure that the sibling has her own hobbies and individual pursuits separate from the person with autism and the family unit.
- Clearly delineate roles for the sibling within the household in terms of what are parents' worries or responsibilities (e.g., finances, planning holidays, organizing the household routines) and what are appropriate responsibilities for her (e.g., keeping her room neat, having her backpack packed ready for school, completing her homework).
- Teach the sibling ways to overcome any feelings of shame or embarrassment about her brother or sister with autism, i.e., brave thoughts to use, activities to engage in to distract her from these feelings, key people she can talk to about feelings of embarrassment.
- Brainstorm special activities for the sibling to engage in with one or both parents as her own "special time" with them (e.g., walks, bike rides, board games, cooking, drawing, reading, movies, swimming).

In Summary

- Parents of a child or children with an ASD can be more vulnerable to experiencing anxiety difficulties than parents of children who do not have an ASD.
- It is important to support anxious parents so that they can, in turn, support their family more effectively. Options for support for parents include:
  - Relaxation skills
  - Seeking individual treatment with a mental health professional
  - Attending a parent support group
  - Allocating time that is just for the parent to pursue her own interests or hobbies
  - Remembering to question whether what the parent is worrying about is truly problematic or "normal" for her child's development
- CBT for anxious parents of children with autism might focus on:
  - Education about anxiety
  - Teaching relaxation skills
  - Working on any unhelpful cognitions around their parenting ability as well as any other worries they have about their daily living activities
  - Graded exposure tasks that relate to their worries, not their child's worries.
- Sometimes parents resist accessing anxiety support. It is important to provide parents with information about anxiety and its impact so that they can ultimately come to their own decision about seeking assistance rather than having it forced upon them.
- Siblings of people with autism can be vulnerable to anxiety because of the pressures of living with a brother or sister with special needs.
- Siblings require special attention and time to ensure that they develop self-confidence and resilience.

Epilogue:
Where Are They Now?

To conclude, the following is an update on some of the families referred to at the start of each chapter. It is so important to have follow-up with or feedback from families to see what, if any, progress is being made with the skills or strategies they have been working on. Below is a brief summary from some of them:

Justin and the Malouf Family

Recap

Justin is the bright but socially anxious high school student with high functioning autism who was going to great lengths to avoid social interaction with his peers. He would retreat to the school library, ask his mother to pick him up from school, or simply avoid going to school for fear of socializing. Justin feared people laughing at him or thinking he was foolish stating, "I'd rather be sliced up than have other people laugh at me."

Outcome

After his diagnosis, Justin began working with me on a weekly basis using a cognitive behavior therapy (CBT) approach to target his social anxiety and worries. Meetings were also held in consultation with his parents and his school teachers to outline strategies for support for him at home and school. By the end of therapy Justin was attending school without difficulty on a daily basis. He had joined a book writing club. According to Justin and his school teachers, he had also developed friendships with three students whom he spent time with both during and outside of school. Justin's application to his studies also seemed to improve. When I spoke with Justin's school psychologist recently, he informed me that Justin now ranks within the top fifteen students in his grade (the school is a selective and academically rigorous high school). Interestingly, Justin is planning on studying psychology at college once he completes his final exams at the end of this year!

Karl and the Potter Family

Recap

Karl was the student who, despite a clean bill of health, frequently made up health-related excuses as to why he could not participate on the playground, for example that he was still recovering from a broken arm (that occurred almost six months prior), or that he was feeling unwell and thought the library might be more relaxing in case it got too hot on the playground and he became faint. Karl had a tendency to catastrophize how bad the playground experience might be. Consequently, Karl was spending most of his recess time in the library, away from his school peers.

Outcome

As mentioned in Chapter 2, I had a consultation with Karl's school. With Karl's help, we developed a plan to slowly integrate Karl into spending time on the playground as well as in the library. Visual and reward systems were used to support and reinforce Karl's bravery and efforts to socialize with his classmates. Karl also attended some individual sessions with me to work on his catastrophic thinking about the dangers of socializing and his tendency to misinterpret social interaction with his peers.

Currently, Karl spends two lunch times per week in the library and the rest on the playground with his peers. Recently, he has developed two friendships with students in his class. Karl and his mother continue to work on his social skills. His tendency to catastrophize how bad a social experience might be has reduced; however, he does need reminding from his parents and school teachers about more helpful ways to think about socializing.

Mitchell

Recap

Mitchell was anxious about winning and losing. He was vigilant regarding the mascot reward system used in his class and whether or not he ended up the winner. If he did not, he would have a "meltdown" and, at times, run out of his classroom.

Outcome

Mitchell's mother, his class teacher, special education coordinator, the speech pathologist from our center, and myself all met at Mitchell's school to discuss suitable reward and behavior management systems for him. Rather than a delayed system, whereby Mitchell earns points that may or may not allow him to take the class mascot home for the weekend, we agreed to establish a more immediate reward system within the classroom. Consequently, Mitchell earns a range of rewards such as stickers, table points, praise, extra computer time, or allocation of a special job for his efforts in class.

Simultaneously, Mitchell started behavior therapy with a psychologist in our center to work through "exposing" him to situations where he might not always win/be the best/be the first, and at the same time teach him relaxation skills and some "helpful thoughts" to use to cope. Mitchell has been able to cope with losing games within his home and not being chosen first in his class. He continues to access individual therapy to work on more challenging situations where he feels he is losing or not doing as well as he might predict.

Angela and Nathan, Parents of Thomas

Recap

Angela and Nathan were fraught with anxiety regarding what kind of school placement would be best for Thomas. They believed that he would be best supported within a fully inclusive school; however, the school was cautious about this prospect. They wanted help regarding how best to manage his transition from a special school into a fully inclusive environment.

Outcome

Thomas was eventually placed in a mainstream school. The school professionals, Angela, Nathan, and I all met to develop a gradual attendance plan for Thomas. The aim was to gradually expose him to the new school environment as well as gradually desensitize his teacher to any fear regarding the experience of working with a child with autism.

Regular review meetings have occurred at the school to establish and refine goals for Thomas's learning and support. Thomas and his parents also attend monthly sessions with a psychologist from our center to work on home management strategies, including ways for the parents to manage Thomas's challenging behavior and anxiety. Now, Thomas is attending school for full days without disruption or difficulty. He recently performed in both a school assembly and play.

Andrew and the Boyce Family

Recap

Andrew was refusing to eat any food that he believed was not prepared for him by his mother. He would ask repeated questions regarding food preparation until he felt satisfied that his mother had made his food. Andrew's rigidity around eating was taking its toll on his mother and on the relationship between his parents as they argued over how best to address his anxiety.

Outcome

Andrew's mother has been working on a weekly basis with a psychologist and a behavior therapist to help address Andrew's anxiety about eating food that anyone other than she has prepared. Together, they've developed a set of goals to work on to gradually expose Andrew to food prepared by others. Some of the goals include Andrew's father touching food when his mother is preparing it. Further up the "stepladder" are goals such as coping when his father prepares one half of his meal and his mother the other half.

Andrew's anxieties regarding food are long-standing and quite entrenched. Although he is making progress in accepting his father's involvement in meal preparation, it will take some time for him to feel comfortable with a range of other people preparing meals for him, which is the final goal for him. Andrew's family will likely continue to benefit from professional support until they are able to achieve this final goal.

Tim and the Rossen Family

Recap

Tim was growing anxious about attending high school the following year. He was frequently worrying about whether or not he would be able to cope with the teachers, the larger environment, the workload, and the other students. His anticipatory anxiety about high school was becoming so intense that he was losing sleep and his appetite because of worry. Tim's parents were seeking the best possible treatment for him to manage his anxiety. They came to me for advice about which treatment options to pursue.

Outcome

After discussion with me about the pros and cons of various anxiety treatments, Tim's parents chose two approaches to try to reduce his social anxiety and his fears about high school. First, they sought support from a medical specialist who assessed Tim and suggested a restricted diet along with the introduction of certain supplements and vitamins to help manage his anxiety. Second, they chose to take Tim to see a psychologist in their local area to teach him relaxation skills. The psychologist also worked on Tim's sleep difficulties, using relaxation skills to help him reduce worry before bed.

After approximately six months, Tim's parents and I met to review his progress. They reported that they found it too hard to maintain a special diet for him and had ceased the dietary intervention approximately eight weeks after starting it. They also said that the costs involved were too high. Furthermore, they did not notice any shifts in Tim's negative thoughts about attending high school when he was on the diet. Rather, they indicated that the more Tim attended high school, the more he was able to learn for himself that it was not as bad as he anticipated it might be. Finally, they told me that they had benefited from a set of six sessions with a local psychologist. Tim was sleeping better and had been using relaxation skills daily before attending school. Tim will soon complete a major series of high school exams and seems to be coping well with balancing the demands of study, socializing, different teachers, and various assignments.

Jeremy and the Fraser Family

Recap

Jeremy had significant anxiety regarding toileting as well as a range of other phobias including a fear of night time, going to school, leaving the house, and bees. His parents were seeking a CBT-based intervention to assist in managing Jeremy's anxiety about toileting and the other phobias. Jeremy was wearing Pull-Ups diapers at school and at home.

Outcome

As mentioned in Chapter 8, with CBT intervention, Jeremy reached a stage where he was successfully using the toilet at home for both bowel and bladder movements but not at school. He was worried about using normal underwear at school instead of Pull-Ups diapers. Therefore, after consultation with the school, his teacher agreed to support the idea of a gradual and slow exposure process for Jeremy in reducing his use of Pull-Ups and increasing time periods for wearing "normal" underwear. These "no Pull-Ups" time periods were then slowly extended as Jeremy attained success. With help from the classroom teacher, the school psychologist, and myself, Jeremy continued to work on exposure steps toward toileting in the school bathrooms. A visual cue of a ladder with steps to represent each toileting goal or exposure task and related rewards for his efforts was prepared. A brave thinking book containing a range of helpful thoughts about using the toilet was also established for Jeremy's reference whenever he was preparing to use the toilet.

Jeremy's parents are now working on extending his confidence wearing underwear and using toilets beyond his home (e.g., public toilets and toilets in other people's homes). They continue to report positive outcomes.

The Turner Family

Recap

Bradley Turner was growing increasingly frustrated and anxious regarding his brother, Mark, who has autism. He was feeling as though the family would never overcome Mark's social difficulties and that he would always be burdened with Mark's circumstances. He also felt unsupported by his parents, whom he believed were spending a disproportionate amount of time with Mark rather than him because of Mark's special needs.

Outcome

Bradley, Mark, and their parents attended approximately eight bi-weekly sessions to work on the problems they were having in managing

Mark's tantrums and reducing Bradley's anxiety and frustration about living with a sibling with autism. During these sessions, we established some structured and equitable behavior management approaches for the parents that all family members agreed to and, therefore, took more responsibility for. For example, disciplining both boys equally and avoiding entering into debates with them regarding "who started what first." Simultaneously, we focused on ways that the parents could re-allocate their time more equitably between Mark and Bradley. Both boys were put in charge of creating a list of activities and interests that they could pursue on their own as well as a list of activities that they could complete together as a "team." Reward systems were then set in place to reinforce their "team work." Bradley was also placed in charge of developing a list of helpful thoughts for him to refer to when he was feeling worried about Mark's difficulties and the impact on the family. Bradley and Mark worked together on a similar (but more visually depicted) list for Mark to use during board games when he needed positive thoughts to cope with losing a game.

Like all families, the Turners continue to experience some conflict between the two boys from time to time. However, all family members now report having better quality relationships with each other and feeling less anxious about the future.

<table>
<tr><td>**Appendix
A**</td><td># Assessment Measures
for Anxiety</td></tr>
</table>

Websites with free measures to assess anxiety:

- Spence Child Anxiety Scale (SCAS; Spence, 1998)
  http://www.scaswebsite.com
  *Parent- and self-report scales for assessing anxiety
  from preschool and beyond.*

- Children's Automatic Thoughts Scale
  (CATS; Schniering & Rapee, 2002)
  http://www.psy.mq.edu.au/CEH/CATS.html
  *Self-report measure that looks at anxious self-talk and
  negative self-statements. The CATS is designed for children
  and adolescents aged eight to seventeen.*

- Strengths and Difficulties Questionnaire
  (SDQ; Goodman, 1997)
  http://www.sdqinfo.org
  *Parent- and teacher-report measures to assess behav-
  iors, including anxiety, in three- to sixteen-year-olds.*

Anxiety assessment measures that can be purchased from test publishers:

- The Anxiety Disorders Interview Schedule for DMS-IV
  (ADIS; Albano & Silverman, 1996)
  *The ADIS is a structured interview schedule for use by
  mental health professionals.*
  Available from:
  ❑ Oxford University Press—http://www.us.oup.com

- The Revised Children's Manifest Anxiety Scale (RC-MAS-2; Reynolds & Richmond, 2008)

  Self-report measure that assesses anxiety in people six to nineteen years of age.

  Available from:
  - Western Psychological Services—http://www.wpspublish.com
  - Pearson—http://www.pearsonpsychcorp.com.au
  - ACER—http://www.acer.edu.au

- Beck Anxiety Inventory (BAI; Beck, Epstein, Brown & Steer, 1988)

  Self-report measure that assesses anxiety in people seventeen to eighty years of age.

  Available from:
  - Pearson—http://www.pearsonassessments.com

- Developmental Behaviour Checklist (DBC; Einfeld & Tonge, 1995)

  The DBC is used to assess behavior and emotional problems in people four to eighteen years of age with developmental and intellectual disabilities. The questionnaire can be completed by parents, other primary caregivers, or teachers.

  Available from:
  - Western Psychological Services—http://www.wpspublish.com

- Child Behavior Checklist (CBCL; Achenbach, 1991)

  The CBCL has parent- and teacher-report forms for use regarding children from infancy to eighteen years of age.

  Available from:
  - Australian Council for Educational Research (ACER)—http://www.acer.edu.au

Adele Faber and Elaine Mazlish website
http://www.fabermazlish.com
    Wide range of resources on how to communicate with children to help them learn how to deal with feelings including anxiety.

Anxiety Disorders Association of America (ADAA)
http://www.adaa.org
    National nonprofit organization solely dedicated to informing the public and healthcare professionals about anxiety disorders, their symptoms, and treatment approaches.

Centre for Emotional Health
http://www.psy.mq.edu.au/CEH
    Eminent research center in Australia focusing on the understanding, treatment, and prevention of anxiety, depression, and related mental health problems. Provides a wide range of evidence-based questionnaires, books, and resources on anxiety management including the internationally acclaimed "Cool Kids" anxiety treatment program.

The Gottman Relationship Institute
http://www.gottman.com
    Excellent resources for parents on Emotion Coaching and developing resilient children.

TEACCH (Treatment and Education of Autistic and related Communication-handicapped Children)

http://www.teacch.com

Excellent information and resources regarding structured teaching and the use of visual supports and visual work systems.

Worry Wise Kids

http://www.worrywisekids.org

Provides parents, educators, and mental health professionals with comprehensive, user-friendly information on the full range of anxiety disorders.

Helpful Books and Resources

Resources to Build Emotional Awareness

Mind Reading: An Interactive Guide to Emotions (Jessica Kingsley Ltd., 2003)
http://www.jkp.com/mindreading
   A good tool for developing emotion recognition and awareness in people with an ASD.

Attwood, T. (2004). *Exploring Feelings: Cognitive Behavior Therapy to Manage Anxiety*. Arlington, Texas: Future Horizons Inc.
   A good program to assist people with an ASD in learning to control emotions. The structured program includes a workbook for the child with activities and information to explore the specific feelings of being happy, relaxed, anxious, or angry.

Buggey, T. (2009). *Seeing is Believing: Video Self-Modeling for People with Autism and Other Developmental Disabilities*. Bethesda, MD: Woodbine House.
   Teaches parents and teachers how to use video self-modeling to help children with autism acquire and improve skills, including recognizing facial expression, fostering communication and social interaction, and controlling tantrums.

Emotion Coaching Resources

Faber, A. & Mazlish, E. (1980). *How to Talk So Kids Will Listen & Listen So Kids Will Talk*. New York, NY: Avon Books Inc.
   This book provides helpful information for parents about empathy and emotion coaching to help them help their children regulate their emotional responses.

Gottman, J. (1997). *Raising an Emotionally Intelligent Child: The Heart of Parenting*. New York, NY: Fireside.

   A great resource for parents and caregivers. The book explains how to coach children to regulate their emotions in order to increase their self-confidence and develop better social relationships.

Self-help Guides

Barlow, D. H. & Craske, M. G. (2007). *Mastering Your Anxiety and Panic: Workbook*. Fourth Edition. New York, NY: Oxford.

   Useful, step-by-step guide for adults to learn skills to manage their own anxiety difficulties.

Huebner, D. (2006). *What to Do When You Worry Too Much: A Kid's Guide to Overcoming Anxiety*. Washington, DC: Magination Press.

   Guides children and parents through a wide range of techniques to manage and reduce anxiety.

Rapee, R., Wignall, A., Spence, S., Cobham, V. & Lyneham, H. (2008). *Helping Your Anxious Child: A Step-by-Step Guide for Parents*. Second Edition. Oakland, CA: New Harbinger Publications, Inc.

   An excellent guide for parents, providing them with many practical skills to help their child overcome anxiety.

Anxiety Prevention for Children

Chalfant, A. M. & Kyngdon, J. C. D. (2008). *Wally the Worried Wallaby in Dog-Gone Trouble*. Sydney, NSW: Annie's Centre.

   The book aims to teach anxious children and their parents skills to manage worries. It also aims to teach parents how to prevent anxiety from developing in their children. A separate parent guide contains ten activities for parents to complete with their child to teach bravery and resilience and to conquer fears and worries. The book and parent guide are available from Annie's Centre: http://www.anniescentre.com.

Webster, A. (2011). *Off We Go to the Dentist*. Bethesda, MD: Woodbine House.

   Children's book intended to help anxious children visualize and practice routines so as to help alleviate their fears about what's going to happen at the dentist.

Webster, A. (2011). *Off We Go to the Grocery Store*. Bethesda, MD: Woodbine House.
    Children's book intended to help anxious children visualize and practice routines so as to help alleviate their fears about what's going to happen on a visit to the grocery store.

Webster, A. (2011). *Off We Go for a Haircut*. Bethesda, MD: Woodbine House.
    Children's book intended to help anxious children visualize and practice routines so as to help alleviate their fears about what's going to happen when they get a haircut.

Resource for Improving Social Skills in Children with an ASD

Weiss, M. J. & Harris, S. L. (2001). *Reaching Out, Joining In: Teaching Social Skills to Young Children with Autism*. Bethesda, MD: Woodbine House.
    A practical and accessible guide describing activities and strategies to use at home and school to foster basic interactive play skills and teach children with autism to recognize social cues and engage in social conversation.

Resource for Determining the Function of a Behavior

Glasberg, B. A. (2006). *Functional Behavior Assessment for People with Autism: Making Sense of Seemingly Senseless Behavior*. Bethesda, MD: Woodbine House.
    Step-by-step instructions for conducting a functional behavior assessment (FBA) to determine the reason for problem behaviors such as aggression, noncompliance, and repetitive actions.

Resources for Teachers

Fein, D. & Dunn, M. A. (2007). *Autism in Your Classroom: A General Educator's Guide to Students with Autism Spectrum Disorders*. Bethesda, MD: Woodbine House.
    Clinical and classroom experience is shared, providing general education teachers who work with children with autism a variety of teaching strategies, as well as ways to manage behavior and sensory issues, and to work on social skills.

Packer, L. E. & Pruitt, S. K. (2010). *Challenging Kids, Challenged Teachers: Teaching Students with Tourette's, Bipolar Disorder, Executive Dysfunction, OCD, ADHD, and More*. Bethesda, MD: Woodbine House.

Experienced authors explain how these conditions, including Asperger's disorder, affect kids' learning and behavior, and offer dozens of proven, practical teaching strategies that can help improve academics, social skills, and emotional stability.

Resource for Dealing with Sensory Issues

Lashno, M. (2010). *Mixed Signals: Understanding and Treating Your Child's Sensory Processing Issues*. Bethesda, MD: Woodbine House.

Helps parents and teachers understand the reasons why some children with autism overreact or underreact to sensory input. Explains how different treatment approaches work and what sensory strategies can help kids accomplish everyday tasks.

Resources for Using Visual Supports and Communication Systems

Bondy, A. & Frost, L. (2011). *A Picture's Worth: PECS and Other Visual Communication Strategies, 2nd Ed*. Bethesda, MD: Woodbine House.

Presents in detail the groundbreaking Picture Exchange Communication System (PECS) that allows a child to use picture to express his needs and desires without prompting for another person.

Cohen, M. J. & Sloan, D. L. (2007). *Visual Supports for People with Autism: A Guide for Parents and Professionals*. Bethesda, MD: Woodbine House.

Learn to create and use visual supports—any pictorial, graphic, or scheduling aid—for use with children with autism. For use at home and in school, these tools improve learning in these areas: language, memory, sequential skills, attention, motivation, and social skills.

McClannahan, L. E. & Krantz, P. J. (2010). *Activity Schedules for Children with Autism: Teaching Independent Behavior*. Bethesda, MD: Woodbine House.

Provides tips on using activity schedules to organize all aspects of a person's daily activities to get tasks completed, keep him engaged and attentive, and to foster social interaction.

Resources for Siblings

Harris, S. L. & Glasberg, B. A. (2003). *Siblings of Children with Autism: A Guide for Families*. Bethesda, MD: Woodbine House.

This family guide explores the basics of sibling relationships and the complexities that surface in families of children with autism. It covers how to explain autism to siblings, get siblings to share their feelings and concerns, master the family balancing act, and foster play between siblings.

Comprehensive CBT Anxiety Treatment Programs for Professionals

As discussed in Chapter 8, a comprehensive cognitive behavior therapy (CBT) program for treating anxiety difficulties in people with an ASD now exists. The details of the child, parent, and therapist manuals for the program are noted below. They are available from the Centre for Emotional Health (http://www.psy.mq.edu.au/CEH) or from Annie's Centre (http://www.anniescentre.com).

Chalfant, A., Lyneham, H. J., Rapee, R. M. & Carroll, L. (2011). *The Cool Kids® Child Anxiety Program: Autism Spectrum Disorders Adaptation. Therapist Manual*. Centre for Emotional Health, Macquarie University: Sydney.

Chalfant, A., Lyneham, H. J., Rapee, R. M. & Carroll, L. (2011). *The Cool Kids® Child Anxiety Program: Autism Spectrum Disorders Adaptation. Children's Workbook*. Centre for Emotional Health, Macquarie University: Sydney.

Lyneham, H. J., Chalfant, A., Rapee, R. M. & Carroll, L. (2011). *The Cool Kids® Child Anxiety Program: Autism Spectrum Disorder Adaptation. Parent's Workbook*. Centre for Emotional Health, Macquarie University: Sydney.

References

Achenbach, T. M. (1991). *Integrative Guide to the 1991 CBCL/4-18, YSR, and TRF Profiles*. Burlington, VT: University of Vermont, Department of Psychology.

Albano, A. M. & Kendall, P. C. (2002). Cognitive behavioural therapy for children and adolescents with anxiety disorders: clinical research advances. *International Review of Psychiatry, 14*, 129-134.

Albano, A. M. & Silverman, W. K. (1996). *Anxiety Disorders Interview Schedule for DSM-IV: Child Version. Clinical Manual*. San Antonio, TX: Psychological Corporation.

American Psychiatric Association. (2000). *Diagnostic and Statistical Manual of Mental Disorders (4th ed. Text revision)*. Washington, DC: American Psychiatric Association.

Anderson, J. C. (1994). Epidemiological issues. In T. H. Ollendick, N. J. King & W. Yule (Eds.), *International Handbook of Phobic and Anxiety Disorders in Children and Adolescents, Issues in Clinical Child Psychology* (pp. 43-65). New York, NY: Plenum Press.

Barlow, D. H. & Craske, M. G. (2007). *Mastering Your Anxiety and Panic: Workbook. Fourth Edition*. New York, NY: Oxford.

Barrett, P. M., Dadds, M. R. & Rapee, R. M. (1996). Family treatment of childhood anxiety: A controlled trial. *Journal of Consulting and Clinical Psychology, 64*, 333-342.

Barrett, P. M., Duffy, A. L., Dadds, M. R. & Rapee, R. M. (2001). Cognitive-behavioral treatment of anxiety disorders in children: Long-term (6 year) follow-up. *Journal of Consulting and Clinical Psychology, 69*, 135-141.

Barrett, P. M. & Turner, C. M. (2001). Prevention of anxiety symptoms in primary school children: Preliminary results from a universal school-based trial. *British Journal of Clinical Psychology, 40*, 399-410.

Barrett, P. M. & Turner, C. M. (2004). Prevention strategies. In T. L. Morris & J. S. March (Eds.). *Anxiety Disorders in Children and Adolescents* (pp. 371-387). New York, NY: Guilford.

Beck, A. T. (1976). *Cognitive Therapy and the Emotional Disorders.* Oxford, England: International Universities Press.

Beck, A. T., Emery, G. & Greenberg, R. L. (2005). *Anxiety Disorders and Phobias: A Cognitive Perspective.* New York, NY: Basic Books.

Beck, A. T., Epstein, N., Brown, G. & Steer, R. A. (1988). An inventory for measuring clinical anxiety: Psychometric properties. *Journal of Consulting and Clinical Psychology, 56*, 893-897.

Beebe, D. W. & Risi, S. (2003). Treatment of adolescents and young adults with high-functioning Autism or Asperger syndrome. In M. A. Reinecke, F. M. Dattilio & A. Freeman (Eds.), *Cognitive Therapy with Children and Adolescents: A Casebook for Clinical Practice, 2nd ed.* (pp. 369-401). New York, NY: Guilford.

Bellini, S. (2004). Social skill deficits and anxiety in high-functioning adolescents with autism spectrum disorders. *Focus on Autism and Other Developmental Disabilities, 19*, 78-86.

Ben-Sasson, A., Cermak, S. A., Orsmond, G. I., Tager-Flusberg, H., Kadlec, M. B. & Carter, A. S. (2008). Sensory clusters of toddlers with autism spectrum disorders: Differences in affective symptoms. *Journal of Child Psychology and Psychiatry, 49*, 817-825.

Bhardwaj, A., Agarwal, V. & Sitholey, P. (2005). Asperger's disorder with co-morbid separation anxiety disorder: A case report. *Journal of Autism and Developmental Disorders, 35*, 135–136.

Braconnier, A. (1983). Autistic anxiety: Psychoanalytic approach. *Neuropsychiatrie de L'Enfance et de L'Adolescence, 31,* 255-256.

Buitelaar, J. K., Van der Gaag, J. & Van der Hoeven, J. (1998). Buspirone in the management of anxiety and irritability in children with pervasive developmental disorders: Results of an open-label study. *Journal of Clinical Psychiatry, 59,* 56–59.

Cannon, W. (1929). *Bodily Changes in Pain, Hunger, Fear, and Rage.* New York, NY: Appleton.

Chalfant, A. M. & Kyngdon, J. C. D. (2008). *Wally the Worried Wallaby in Dog-Gone Trouble.* Sydney, NSW: Annie's Centre.

Chalfant, A., Lyneham, H. J., Rapee, R. M. & Carroll, L. (2011). *The Cool Kids® Child Anxiety Program: Autism Spectrum Disorder Adaptation. Children's Workbook.* Centre for Emotional Health, Macquarie University: Sydney.

Chalfant, A., Lyneham, H. J., Rapee, R. M. & Carroll, L. (2011). *The Cool Kids® Child Anxiety Program: Autism Spectrum Disorder Adaptation. Therapist Manual.* Centre for Emotional Health, Macquarie University: Sydney.

Chalfant, A., Rapee, R. & Carroll, L. (2006). Treating anxiety disorders in children with high-functioning autism spectrum disorders: A controlled trial. *Journal of Autism and Developmental Disorders, 33,* 283-298.

Chambless, D. & Hollon, S. D. (1998). Defining empirically supported therapies. *Journal of Consulting and Clinical Psychology, 6,* 7-18.

Clark, D. M. & Wells, A. (1995). A cognitive model of social phobia. In R. G. Heimberg, M. R. Liebowitz, D. A. Hope & F. R. Schneier (Eds.). *Social Phobia: Diagnosis, Assessment, and Treatment* (pp. 69-93). New York, NY: Guilford.

Craske, M. G. & Barlow, D. H. (1991). Contributions of cognitive psychology to assessment and treatment of anxiety. In Martin, P. R. (Ed). *Handbook of Behavior Therapy and Psychological Science: An Integrative Approach.* Elmsford, NY: Pergamon Press.

Drake, K. L. & Kearney, C. A. (2008). Child anxiety sensitivity and family environment as mediators of the relationship between parent psychopathology, parent anxiety sensitivity, and child anxiety. *Journal of Psychopathology and Behavioral Assessment, 30*, 79-86.

Einfeld, S. L. & Tonge, B. J. (1995). The Developmental Behavior Checklist: The development and validation of an instrument to assess behavioral and emotional disturbance in children and adolescents with mental retardation. *Journal of Autism and Developmental Disorders, 25*, 81-104.

Erikson, E. H. (1950). *Childhood and Society.* New York, NY: Norton & Company Inc.

Faber, A. & Mazlish, E. (1980). *How to Talk So Kids Will Listen & Listen So Kids Will Talk.* New York, NY: Avon Books Inc.

Fombonne, E., Simmons, H., Ford, T., Meltzer, H. & Goodman, R. (2001). Prevalence of pervasive developmental disorders in the British Nationwide Survey of Child Mental Health. *Journal of the American Academy of Child and Adolescent Psychiatry, 40*, 820-827.

Frith, U. (1989). *Autism: Explaining the Enigma.* Oxford, England: Blackwell.

Gal, E., Cermak, S. A. & Ben-Sasson, A. (2007). Sensory processing disorders in children with autism: Nature, assessment, and intervention. In R. L. Gabriels & D. E. Hill (Eds.). *Growing Up with Autism: Working with School-age Children and Adolescents* (pp. 95-123). New York, NY: Guilford Press.

Gar, N. S. & Hudson, J. L. (2008). An examination of the interactions between mothers and children with anxiety disorders. *Behaviour Research and Therapy, 46*, 1266-1274.

Gar, N. S., Hudson, J. L. & Rapee, R. M. (2005). Family factors and the development of anxiety disorders. In J. L. Hudson & R. M. Rapee (Eds.). *Psychopathology and the Family* (pp. 125-145). New York, NY: Elsevier Science.

Ghaziuddin, M. (2002). Asperger syndrome: Associated psychiatric and medical conditions. *Focus on Autism and Other Developmental Disabilities, 17,* 138-144.

Gillot, A., Furniss, F. & Walter, A. (2001). Anxiety in high-functioning children with autism. *Autism, 5,* 277-286.

Goodman, R. (1997). The strengths and difficulties questionnaire: A research note. *Journal of Child Psychology and Psychiatry, 38,* 581-586.

Gottman, J. (1997). *Raising an Emotionally Intelligent Child.* New York, NY: Fireside.

Hanson, E., Kalish, L. A., Bunce, E., Curtis, C., McDaniel, S., Ware, J. & Petry, J. (2007). Use of complementary and alternative medicine among children diagnosed with autism spectrum disorder. *Journal of Autism and Developmental Disorders, 37,* 628-636.

Happé, F. G. E. (1994). Annotation: Current psychological theories of autism: The "Theory of Mind" account and rival theories. *Journal of Child Psychology and Psychiatry, 35,* 215-229.

Happé, F. & Frith, U. (2006). The weak coherence account: Detail focused cognitive style in autism spectrum disorders. *Journal of Autism and Developmental Disorders, 36,* 5-25.

Harrison Elder, J., Shankar, M., Shuster, J., Theriaque, D., Burns, S. & Sherrill, L. (2006). The gluten-free, casein-free diet in autism: Results of a preliminary double blind clinical trial. *Journal of Autism and Developmental Disorders, 36,* 413-420.

Heinemann, E. (1999). Psychoanalytic therapy with an autistic young man: A discussion of Frances Tustin's theories. In J. De Groef & E. Heinemann (Eds.), *Psychoanalysis and Mental Handicap* (pp. 23-40). London, England: Free Association Books.

Hudson, J. L. & Rapee, R. M. (2004). From anxious temperament to disorder: An etiological model of generalized anxiety disorder. In R. G. Heimberg, C. L. Turk & D. S. Mennin (Eds.), *Generalized Anxiety Disorder: Advances in Research and Practice* (pp. 51-76). New York, NY: Guilford Press.

Jacobson, E. (1938). *Progressive Relaxation (2nd ed.)*. Oxford, England: University of Chicago Press.

Johnson, S. M. & Hollander, E. (2003). Evidence that eicosapentaenic acid is effective in treating autism. *Journal of Clinical Psychiatry, 64*, 848–849.

Keller, M. B., Lavoir, P., Wunder, J., Beardslee, W. R., Schwarts, E. & Roth, J. (1992). Chronic course of anxiety disorders in children and adolescents. *Journal of the American Academy of Child and Adolescent Psychiatry, 31*, 100-110.

Kendall, P. C. (1985). Toward a cognitive-behavioural model of child psychopathology and a critique of related interventions. *Journal of Abnormal Child Psychology, 13*, 357-372.

Kendall, P. C. (1994). Treating anxiety disorders in children: Results of a randomized clinical trial. *Journal of Consulting and Clinical Psychology, 62*, 100-110.

Kendall, P. C., Flannery-Schroeder, E., Panichelli-Mindel, S., Southam-Gerow, M., Henin, A. & Warman, M. (1997). Therapy for youths with anxiety disorders: A second randomized clinical trial. *Journal of Consulting and Clinical Psychology, 65*, 366-380.

Kendall, P. C., Safford, S., Flannery-Schroeder, E. & Webb, A. (2004). Child anxiety treatment: Outcomes in adolescence and impact on substance use and depression at 7.4 year follow-up. *Journal of Consulting and Clinical Psychology, 72*, 276-287.

Klin, A., Saulnier, C. A., Sparrow, S. S., Cicchetti, D. V., Volkmar, F. R. & Lord, C. (2007). Social and communication abilities and disabilities in higher functioning individuals with autism spectrum disorders: The Vineland and the ADOS. *Journal of Autism and Developmental Disorders, 37*, 748-759.

Lehmkuhl, H. D., Storch, E. A., Bodfish, J. W. & Geffken, G. R. (2008). Brief report: Exposure and response prevention for obsessive compulsive disorder in a 12-year-old with autism. *Journal of Autism and Developmental Disorders, 38*, 977-981.

Lewis, M. H. & Bodfish, J. W. (1998). Repetitive behavior disorders in autism. *Mental Retardation and Developmental Disabilities, 4*, 80-89.

Lyneham, H. J., Chalfant, A., Rapee, R. M. & Carroll, L. (2011). *The Cool Kids® Child Anxiety Program: Autism Spectrum Disorders Adaptation. Parent's Workbook*. Centre for Emotional Health, Macquarie University: Sydney.

McGovern, C. W. & Sigman, M. (2005). Continuity and change from early childhood to adolescence in autism. *Journal of Child Psychology and Psychiatry, 46*, 401-408.

McLean, C. P. & Anderson E. R. (2009). Brave men and timid women? A review of the gender differences in fear and anxiety. *Clinical Psychology Review, 29*, 496-505.

Mendlowitz, S. L., Manassis, K., Bradley, S., Scapillato, D., Miezitis, S. & Shaw, B. F. (1999). Cognitive-behavioral group treatments in childhood anxiety disorders: The role of parental involvement. *Journal of the American Academy of Child and Adolescent Psychiatry, 38*, 1223-1229.

Mesibov, G. B., Adams, L. & Klinger, L. G. (1997). *Autism: Understanding the Disorder*. New York, NY: Plenum Press.

Mesibov, G.B., Shea, V. & Schopler, E. (2005). *The TEACCH Approach to Autism Spectrum Disorders*. New York, NY: Kluwer Academic/Plenum.

Messer, S. C. & Beidel, D. C. (1994). Psychosocial correlates of childhood anxiety disorders. *Journal of the American Academy of Child and Adolescent Psychiatry, 33*, 975-983.

Muris, P., Steerneman, P., Harald, M., Holdrinet, I. & Meesters, C. (1998). Comorbid anxiety symptoms in children with pervasive developmental disorders. *Journal of Anxiety Disorders, 12*, 387-393.

Nolen-Hoeksema, S. & Jackson, B. (2001). Mediators of the gender difference in rumination. *Psychology of Women Quarterly, 25*, 37–47.

Ozbayrak, K. R. (1997). Sertraline in PDD. *Journal of the American Academy of Child & Adolescent Psychiatry, 36*, 7–8.

Pfeiffer, S. I., Norton, J., Nelson, L. & Shott, S. (1995). Efficacy of vitamin B6 and magnesium in the treatment of autism: A methodology review and summary of outcomes. *Journal of Autism and Developmental Disorders, 25*, 481-493.

Piaget, J. & Inhelder, B. (1973). *Memory and Intelligence.* London, England: Routledge and Kegan Paul.

Piven, J., Chase, G. A., Landa, R., Wzorek, M., Gayle, J., Cloud, D. & Folstein, S. E. (1991). Psychiatric disorders in the parents of autistic individuals. *Journal of the American Academy of Child and Adolescent Psychiatry, 30*, 471-478.

Rapee, R. M. & Heimberg, R. G. (1997). A cognitive-behavioral model of anxiety in social phobia. *Behaviour Research and Therapy, 35*, 741-756.

Rapee, R. M., Wignall, A., Spence, S., Cobham, V. & Lyneham, H. J. (2008). *Helping Your Anxious Child: A Step-by-Step Guide for Parents (2nd ed.).* Oakland, CA: New Harbinger Publications.

Reaven, J. A., Blakeley-Smith, A., Nichols, S., Dasari, M., Flanigan, E. & Hepburn, S. (2009). Cognitive-behavioral group treatment for anxiety symptoms in children with high-functioning autism spectrum disorders: A pilot study. *Focus Autism and Other Developmental Disabilities, 24*, 27-37.

Reaven, J. & Hepburn, S. (2003). Cognitive-behavioral treatment of obsessive-compulsive disorder in a child with asperger syndrome: A case report. *Autism, 7,* 145-164.

Reynolds, C. R. & Richmond, B. O. (1978). What I think and feel: A revised measure of child's manifest anxiety. *Journal of Abnormal Child Psychology, 6*, 271-280.

Ronan, K. R., Kendall, P. C. & Rowe, M. (1994). Negative affectivity in children: Development and validation of a self-statement questionnaire. *Journal of Cognitive Therapy and Research, 18,* 509-528.

Rumsey, J. M., Rapport, J. L. & Sceery, W. R. (1985). Autistic children as adults: Psychiatric, social, and behavioural outcomes. *Journal of the American Academy of Child and Adolescent Psychiatry, 24,* 465-473.

Rutter, M. & Bailey, A. (1994). Thinking and relationships: Mind and brain (some reflections on theory of mind and autism). In Baron-Cohen, S., Tager-Flusberg, H. & Cohen, D. J. (Eds). *Understanding Other Minds: Perspectives from Autism.* New York, NY: Oxford University Press.

Schniering, C. A. & Rapee, R. M. (2002). Development and validation of a measure of children's automatic thoughts: The children's automatic thoughts scale. *Behaviour Research and Therapy, 40,* 1091-1109.

Schteingart, A. (1989). Autism and separation anxiety. *Revue Francaise de Psychanalyse, 53,* 291-296.

Shortt, A. L., Barrett, P. M. & Fox, T. L. (2001). Evaluating the FRIENDS program: A cognitive-behavioral group treatment for anxious children and their parents. *Journal of Clinical Child and Adolescent Psychology, 30,* 525-535.

Silveira, R., Jainer, A. K. & Bates, G. (2004). Fluoxetine treatment of selective mutism in pervasive developmental disorder. *International Journal of Psychiatry in Clinical Practice, 8,* 179–180.

Silverman, W. K., Kurtines, W. M., Ginsburg, G. S., Weems, C. F., Lumpkin, P. W. & Carmichael, D. H. (1999). Treating anxiety disorders in children with group cognitive-behavioral therapy: A randomized clinical trial. *Journal of Consulting and Clinical Psychology, 67,* 995-1003.

Simonoff, E., Pickles, A., Charman, T., Chandler, S., Loucas, T. & Baird, G. (2008). Psychiatric disorders in children with autism spectrum disorders: Prevalence, comorbidity, and associated factors in a population-derived sample. *Journal of the American Academy of Child and Adolescent Psychiatry, 47,* 921-929.

Sivberg, B. (2002). Family system and coping behaviors: A comparison between parents of children with autistic spectrum disorders and parents with non-autistic children. *Autism, 6,* 397-409.

Sofronoff, K., Attwood, T. & Hinton, S. (2005). A randomised controlled trial of a CBT intervention for anxiety in children with Asperger syndrome. *Journal of Child Psychology and Psychiatry, 46,* 1152-1160.

Spence, S. H. (1998). A measure of anxiety symptoms among children. *Behaviour, Research and Therapy, 36,* 545-566.

Steffenburg, S., Gillberg, C. & Steffenburg, U. (1996). Psychiatric disorders in children and adolescents with mental retardation and active epilepsy. *Archives of Neurology, 53,* 904-912.

Sukhodolsky, D. G., Scahill, L., Gadow, K. D., Arnold, L. E., Aman, M. G., McDougle, C. J., MacCracken, J. T., Tierney, E., Williams White, S., Lecavalier, L. & Vitiello, B. (2008). Parent-rated anxiety symptoms in children with pervasive developmental disorders: Frequency and association with core autism symptoms and cognitive functioning. *Journal of Abnormal Child Psychology, 36,* 117-128.

Sze, K. M. & Wood, J. J. (2007). Cognitive behavioral treatment of comorbid anxiety disorders and social difficulties in children with high-functioning autism: A case report. *Journal of Contemporary Psychotherapy, 37,* 133-143.

Tryon, W. W. (2005). Possible mechanisms for why desensitization and exposure therapy work. *Clinical Psychology Review, 25,* 67-95.

Tsai, L. Y. (1999). Pharmacology in autism. *Psychosomatic Medicine, 61,* 651-665.

van der Bruggen, C. O., Stams, G. J. J. M. & Bögels, S. M. (2008). Research review: The relation between child and parent anxiety and parental control: A meta-analytic review. *Journal of Child Psychology and Psychiatry, 49,* 1257-1269.

Verheij, F. & Van Loon, H. (1993). Pervasive developmental disorders not otherwise specified: A developmental-psychopathological approach for the development of made-to-measure treatment planning. *European Journal of Child and Adolescent Psychiatry: Acta Paedopsychiatrica, 55,* 235-242.

White, S. W., Albano, A. M., Johnson, C. R., Kasari, C., Ollendick, T., Klin, A., Oswald, D. & Scahill, L. (2010). Development of a cognitive-behavioral intervention program to treat anxiety and social deficits in teens with high-functioning autism. *Clinical Child and Family Psychology Review, 13,* 77-90.

White, S. W., Oswald, D., Ollendick, T. & Scahill, L. (2009). Anxiety in children and adolescents with autism spectrum disorders. *Clinical Psychology Review, 29,* 216-229.

Wing, L. (1997). The history of ideas on autism. *Autism, 1,* 13-23.

Wolf, L. C., Noh, S., Fisman, S. N. & Speechly, M. (1989). Psychological effects of parenting stress on parents of autistic children. *Journal of Autism and Developmental Disorders, 19,* 157-166.

Wood, J. J., Drahota, A., Sze, K., Har, K., Chiu, A. & Langer, D. A. (2009). Cognitive behavioral therapy for anxiety in children with autism spectrum disorders: A randomized, controlled trial. *Journal of Child Psychology and Psychiatry, 50,* 224-234.

Index

Page numbers in italics indicate figures or tables.

About the Author

Anne Marie Chalfant Psy. D. is a practicing clinical psychologist who specializes in child mental health and developmental disorders. She is the Director of Annie's Centre, a private multi-disciplinary practice in Sydney, Australia that assists children with a range of learning, developmental, and mental health difficulties, as well as their families and the professionals that work with them. She has trained and worked in a variety of settings including public health, non-government organizations, and universities both within Australia and overseas. Currently, she is a lecturer for the University of New South Wales and a clinical supervisor for both the University of New South Wales and the University of Western Sydney, Australia. Anne has presented at both national and international conferences as well as published several articles on anxiety difficulties. Most recently, she co-authored *The Cool Kids Child Anxiety Program: Autism Spectrum Disorders Adaptation* (Chalfant, Lyneham, Rapee & Carroll, 2011). Anne also presents frequently on the topics of parenting and child development on talk-back radio in Sydney.